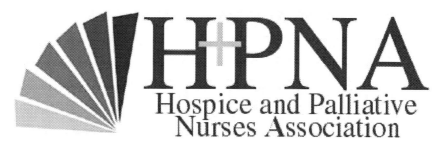

Hospice and Palliative Nursing Assistant Core Curriculum

Editor:
Mary Ersek, PhD, RN, FAAN
Associate Professor
University of Pennsylvania, School of Nursing
Philadelphia, PA

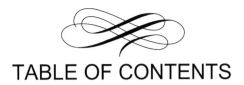

TABLE OF CONTENTS

CONTRIBUTORS
Hospice and Palliative Nursing Assistant Core Curriculum

Patricia Berry, PhD, APRN, GNP-BC, ACHPN®
Associate Professor and Associate Director
University of Utah Hartford Center of Geriatric
Nursing Excellence
University of Utah, College of Nursing
Salt Lake City, UT

Eileen R. Chichin, PhD, RN
Co-Director, Greenberg Center on Ethics
Jewish Home Lifecare
New York, NY

Mary Edwards, RN, CHPN®
Clinical Resource Nurse
Hospice of the Valley
Phoenix, AZ

Mary Ersek, PhD, RN, FAAN
Associate Professor
University of Pennsylvania, School of Nursing
Philadelphia, PA

Barbara Head, PhD, RN, CHPN®, ACSW
Assistant Professor
University of Louisville, School of Medicine
Louisville, KY

Kimberly M. Bergman-Jackson, MSN, RN
Doctoral Student
University of Iowa, College of Nursing
Iowa City, IA

Beth Miller Kraybill, RN, BSN, CHPN®
Research Nurse Coordinator
Swedish Medical Center
Seattle, WA

Judy Lentz, RN, MSN, NHA
CEO
Hospice and Palliative Nurses Association
Pittsburgh, PA

Jeanne Martinez, RN, MPH, CHPN®
Associate Director for Outreach and
Technical Assistance, The EPEC Project
Northwestern University Feinberg School of Medicine
Chicago, IL

Marianne LaPorte Matzo, PhD, APRN, GNP-BC, FAAN
Professor
New Hampshire Community Technical College
Manchester, NH

Jayne E. Pawasauskas, PharmD
Assistant Professor of Clinical Pharmacy
University of Rhode Island
Kingston, RI

Molly Poleto, RN, BSN
Consultant
Delmar, NY

Marty Richards, MSW, LICSW
Consultant on Aging
Port Townsend, WA

Joanne E. Sheldon, MEd, MSN, RN, CHPN®
Education Coordinator for the Hospice Institute
Hospice of the Western Reserve
Cleveland, OH

Sarah A. Wilson, RN, PhD
Associate Professor
Marquette University, College of Nursing
Milwaukee, WI

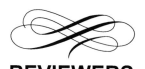

REVIEWERS
Hospice and Palliative Nursing Assistant Core Curriculum

Tami Borneman, RN, MSN, CNS
Senior Research Specialist
Department of Nursing Research & Education
City of Hope National Medical Center
Duarte, CA

Angie Budington, NA, CHPNA®
Nursing Assistant
Richmond, VA

Patrick Coyne, RN, MSN, CS
Clinical Nurse Specialist
Pain Management/Palliative Care
Thomas Palliative Care Unit
Medical College of Virginia Hospitals
Virginia Commonwealth University
Richmond, VA

Mary Edwards, RN, CHPN®
Clinical Resource Nurse
Hospice of the Valley
Phoenix, AZ

Phyllis Freeman, CNA
Certified Nursing Assistant
Franciscan Hospice
Tacoma, WA

Nancy L. Grandovic, RN, BSN, MEd., CHPN®
Assistant Director of Education
Hospice and Palliative Nurses Association
Pittsburgh, PA

Rebecca Kennedy, RN, CRNH
Educator
State of Michigan Program
HCR Manor Care Company
Bloomfield Hills, MI

Pamela Ketzner, RN, MN, CHPN®
Nursing Staff Educator
Franciscan Hospice and Palliative Care
Tacoma. WA

Beth Miller Kraybill BSN, RN, CHPN®
MDiv Program Student
Associated Mennonite Biblical Seminary
Elhart, IN

Judy Lentz, RN, MSN, NHA
CEO
Hospice and Palliative Nurses Association
Pittsburgh, PA

Polly Mazanec, APRN, MSN, AOCN Advanced
Practice Nurse, Palliative Care
Hospice of the Western Reserve
Cleveland, OH

Bridget Montana, APRN, MSN, MBA
Chief Operating Officer
Hospice of the Western Reserve
Cleveland, OH

Dena Jean Sutermaster, RN, MSN, CHPN®
Director of Education/Research
Hospice and Palliative Nurses Association
Pittsburgh, PA

Rose Virani, RNC, BSN, MHA, OCN
Senior Research Specialist
ELNEC Project Director
Department of Nursing Research and Education
City of Hope National Medical Center
Duarte, CA

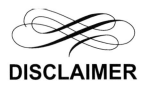

DISCLAIMER

The Hospice and Palliative Nurses Association, its officers and directors and the authors and reviewers of this core curriculum make no claims that buying or studying it will guarantee a passing score on the CHPNA™ Certification examination.

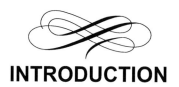

INTRODUCTION

Nursing assistants work in a wide variety of settings, including long-term care, hospitals, home care, and hospice. They play a central role in providing care to patients with progressive, life-limiting illnesses, and in providing care and support for the families of those patients. Since 2003, the Alliance for Excellence in Hospice and Palliative Nursing, comprised of the Hospice and Palliative Nurses Association (HPNA), the National Board for Certification of Hospice and Palliative Nurses (NBCHPN®), and the Hospice and Palliative Nurses Foundation (HPNF), has committed itself to enhancing the education and professional development of nursing assistants.

In 2001, HPNA established nursing assistant membership, an unusual and bold step given that nearly all professional nursing organizations exclude nursing assistants. The Association underscored their support for this group of care providers by publishing a position statement entitled, *The Value of the Nursing Assistant in Palliative Care*. In this document, nurses, administrators, and healthcare organizations are urged to "recognize that care provided by nursing assistants is critical to achieving established goals of care for patients with progressive, life-limiting illness and their families."[1] HPNA also offers a variety of educational opportunities and products intended for nursing assistants. These include the *Nursing Assistant Computerized Educational Program* (NA-CEP), components of the *Generalist Clinical Review Train-the-Trainer Workshop*, and Nursing Assistant teleconferences. NBCHPN® has provided certification for hospice and palliative nursing assistants since 2002. As of 2009, there are over 3,700 dedicated nursing assistants throughout the United States who have achieved this distinction. Every year, the Hospice and Palliative Nurses Foundation offers scholarships for nursing assistants to take the certification examination.

With this revision of the *Hospice and Palliative Nursing Assistant Core Curriculum*, HPNA strives to continue to support nursing assistants and nourish their development as integral members of the palliative care team. Like the first edition, its goal is to enhance the palliative care knowledge base and skills of nursing assistants working in all clinical settings. The principles that guided the development of the first edition of the *Core Curriculum* remain unchanged in this revised edition. We believe that:

- Better educational preparation for Nursing Assistants results in more effective care for patients with progressive, life-limiting illnesses and their families.

- To participate actively in planning and providing quality care to palliative care patients and their families, Nursing Assistants need to possess specialized knowledge and skills.

- Nursing Assistants who are educated and involved in the care of patients with progressive, life-limiting illnesses and their families experience greater job satisfaction, which may in turn decrease job turnover that threatens the quality and consistency of palliative care.

- Although Nursing Assistants do not make decisions about medical therapies or administer medications, they are responsible for observing and reporting the symptoms for which these therapies are given, and for observing and reporting responses to the therapies. In addition, their attitudes towards certain therapies, such as opioids and artificial nutrition, are communicated either directly or indirectly to patients and families. Thus, Nursing Assistants need to be aware of the reasons for instituting or withdrawing therapies and to realize that their attitudes influence patients and families. For this reason, the *Hospice and Palliative Nursing Assistant Core Curriculum* contains information about medical therapies for several symptoms.

This edition contains revised and updated content in every chapter. A new feature has also been added: case studies and questions for each chapter to assess learning and assist in preparation for the certification examination. The *Core Curriculum* is designed to be used either by Nursing Assistants or by educators who prepare Nursing Assistants for clinical practice. We hope that all users of the book will grow in their ability to teach about and provide high-quality, compassionate care to patients with life-limiting illness and their families.

Mary Ersek, PhD, RN, FAAN
Editor, *Hospice and Palliative Nursing Assistant Core Curriculum*

Hospice and Palliative Nurses Association:

Address: One Penn Center West, Suite 229
            Pittsburgh, PA 15276-0100
Phone: 412-787-9301
Fax: 412-787-9305
Email: hpna@hpna.org

Cited References:

1.   Sidwell JC, Ersek M, Kestner M, Miller Kraybill B. *The value of the nursing assistant in palliative care.* Position statement. Approved by the HPNA Board of Directors January 2009. Pittsburgh, PA: Hospice and Palliative Nurses Association; 2009. Available at: http://www.hpna.org/DisplayPage.aspx?Title=Position%20Statements.

CHAPTER 1
OVERVIEW OF HOSPICE AND PALLIATIVE NURSING ASSISTANT PRACTICE

Mary Ersek, PhD, RN, FAAN

Original Authors
Judy Lentz, RN, MSN, NHA, Mary Edwards, RN, CHPN®, and Mary Ersek, RN, PhD, FAAN

"What I do you cannot do; but what you do, I cannot do. The needs are great, and none of us, including me, ever do great things. But we can all do small things, with great love, and together we can do something wonderful."

Mother Teresa, 1910-1997

I. Introduction to Care at the End of Life[1,2]

A. The end of life (EOL) - living and dying well

1. The end of life

   a) Final phase of life - not defined by a time frame, such as six months

   b) Natural part of life

   c) There is an opportunity for personal growth during the process of dying; physical health declines, but many people can experience emotional healing and a sense of peace at the EOL

   d) Profoundly personal experience

2. Dying well

   a) A "good death" is

Dying is a natural part of life.

   i. Free from avoidable distress and suffering

   ii. Reflects patients' and families' goals and values

   iii. Should occur in all care settings, including home, hospital, long-term care facility, prisons

   b) Dying well is a goal that is not always reached because

   i. American society often avoids talking about death and isolates dying people

   ii. Hospice and palliative care services are not always available to patients and families

   iii. Many healthcare providers, including nurses, physicians, nursing assistants, do not know how to provide hospice and palliative care

   iv. Some people do not prepare for death even when seriously ill because they think (wrongly) that a cure is always possible with high technology healthcare

   v. Payment for healthcare services focuses on therapies aimed to cure diseases rather than help people live better with chronic illnesses

      vi.   Comfort care is not standard in all settings because the major goals of treatment and expertise of care providers differs across settings; e.g., focus in acute care often is curing diseases and saving lives; focus in nursing home often is rehabilitation

B.   History of care at the end of life[1,2,3]

  1.   Focus on dying well has developed over the last 10-20 years

  2.   Before the 1900s

     a)   Medicine could not cure most diseases

     b)   Physicians' job was to bring comfort and manage symptoms as much as possible

     c)   Death usually occurred at home

  3.   Early to mid-1900s

     a)   Improved living and working conditions meant that many accidents and diseases were prevented

     b)   Treatment advances, such as the discovery of antibiotics, enabled people to live longer

     c)   Focus of medicine shifted to curing diseases

     d)   Death became a "failure" of medicine to cure the disease

     e)   Most deaths shifted from home setting and occurred in hospitals and other facilities

  4.   1990s to present

     a)   Focus still is very much on curing and technological advances

     b)   Despite these advances, people realize that

        i.   Not all diseases can be cured

        ii.   Death is still a reality

        iii.   More people are living longer with chronic diseases that decrease a person's quality of life

     c)   Studies done in the early 1990s showed that people often received care that kept them alive, but caused great suffering at the EOL; people questioned the focus on high-tech hospital care for patients with incurable illnesses[3]

     d)   Because of these studies, patients are taking a more active role in deciding what happens to them at the end of their lives; many people are choosing comfort care rather than high-tech intensive care when they have a disease that cannot be cured

     e)   In the future, people will continue to live longer, and more people will live with chronic diseases that cause disability

     f)   Healthcare needs to adjust and provide high-quality care for

        i.   Helping people live as well as they can with chronic, life-limiting diseases

ii. Helping people with advanced disease cope with the dying process earlier in the illness experience[4]

C. What is hospice and palliative care?

1. Care provided to patients with serious, life-limiting diseases (in other words, serious illness that cannot be cured) and their families

2. Includes care that is provided at the EOL

3. Features of hospice and palliative care[2,3]

   a) Showing respect for patients' and families' goals, choices, religious and cultural traditions, and spirituality

   b) Giving treatments that match the patients' and families' goals and values

   c) Caring for the whole person, including that person's physical, emotional, social, and spiritual needs

   d) Making the patient's quality of life better by managing symptoms such as pain and loss of appetite

   e) Supporting caregivers, including family members and other people who are close to the patient

   f) Giving care using an interdisciplinary team (IDT) also referred to as an interdisciplinary group (IDG)

   g) Talking openly and honestly about illness and death in a way that respects the needs and values of the patient and family

   h) Providing care to dying patients of all ages, including infants and children

   i) Helping seriously ill patients live as fully as possible until they die

4. Hospice care

   a) System of specialized care that supports patient and families through the final weeks and months of life

   b) Addresses needs of the family and friends following the patient's death (that is, it provides bereavement care)

   c) Provided in many settings, especially in the home and long-term care facilities

   d) Modern hospice care began in 1967 at the St. Christopher's Hospice, London

   e) First modern American hospice: Connecticut Hospice, begun in 1974

   f) Much of hospice care is paid for by the Medicare Hospice Benefit (MHB); Medicare is the United States government health insurance that covers people aged 65 and older, some disabled people who are younger than 65, and any person with very serious kidney failure

   g) Most hospice care is provided by hospice agencies caring for patients in their own homes or in nursing homes

   h) To be eligible for hospice care, a person's doctor has to state that the person is likely to die in 6 months or less

5. Palliative care[3]

   a) A philosophy of care and an organized, highly structured system for delivering care. The goal of palliative care is to prevent and relieve suffering and to

Hospice and Palliative Care is care provided by an interdisciplinary team to patients with a life-limiting illness and their families. This care continues through end-of-life for the patient and provides bereavement care for family and friends.

support the best possible quality of life for patients and their families, regardless of the stage of the disease or the need for other therapies[3]

  b) Affirms life by supporting the patient and family's goals for the future, including their hopes for cure or life-prolongation, as well as their hopes for peace and dignity throughout the course of illness, the dying process and death[3]

  c) Is appropriate for all patients from the time of diagnosis with a life-threatening or life-limiting or debilitating condition, regardless of the patient's age

  d) Care of patients whose disease cannot be cured; focus of care is on pain and symptom management, and on emotional, social, and spiritual needs of patients and families[6]

  e) Care provided by a team of healthcare providers focused on the relief of suffering, and support for the best quality of life for patients facing serious, life-limiting illness, and their families[3]

  f) Palliative care teams work in all types of healthcare delivery system settings; such as hospitals, clinics, emergency departments, nursing homes, home care, assisted living facilities, outpatient, and non-traditional settings

  g) Team collaborates with professional and informal caregivers to ensure coordination, communication, and continuity of care across settings

  h) Similar goals as hospice but palliative care is not limited to EOL care

  i) Palliative care movement began in part as a response to limitations in hospice funding that limit care to the final 6 months of life; because of this limitation, many people with life-limiting chronic diseases, such as Alzheimer's disease and multiple sclerosis, had difficulty meeting the admission criteria

  j) Has evolved into a specialty of its own, but continues to change as healthcare changes

  k) Complements hospice care and provides services earlier in the illness

  l) The National Consensus Project for Quality Palliative Care (NCP) developed *Clinical Practice Guidelines for Quality Palliative Care* as an universal approach to ensure quality palliative care across the nation. Four partnering organizations: Hospice and Palliative Nurses Association (HPNA); American Academy of Hospice and Palliative Medicine (AAHPM); Center to Advance Palliative Care (CAPC); and the National Hospice and Palliative Care Organization (NHPCO)

6. Goals of hospice and palliative care

  a) Achieving the best quality of life for patients and their families when cure is not possible

  b) Providing for a peaceful death, a "good death" as defined by the patient and family

  c) The place of hospice and palliative care in the healthcare system (Figure 1)

> *A major goal of hospice and palliative care is to enhance the quality of life for patients and their families facing, progressive, life-limiting illnesses.*

D. The hospice and palliative care team

  1. Is comprised of the interdisciplinary - team members come from many professional backgrounds or disciplines

  2. Is often referred to as the interdisciplinary team (IDT) or interdisciplinary group (IDG)

3. Team members include
   a) Nurses
   b) Nursing assistants
   c) Chaplain, clergy, and spiritual counselors
   d) Social workers
   e) Physicians
   f) Pharmacists
   g) Dieticians
   h) Physical and occupational therapists
   i) Speech therapists
   j) Volunteers
   k) Bereavement counselors
   l) Healing therapists: art, massage, music, pet therapists
   m) Patient
   n) Family members and other caregivers
   o) Anyone else that can help with care

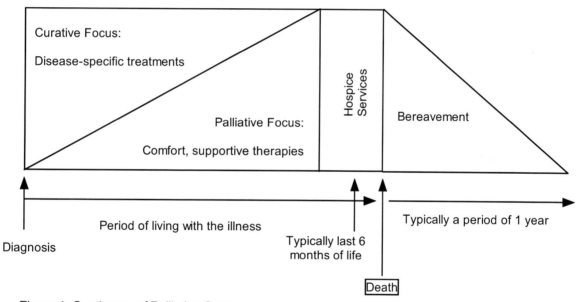

Figure 1. Continuum of Palliative Care

II. Hospice and Palliative Nursing Assistant: Training, Work Setting, and Roles[4]

A. The Nursing Assistant is an important member of the interdisciplinary team

B. Practices under the supervision of a licensed nurse

C. Education obtained through various programs

D. More than 2.5 million Nursing Assistants in many settings; over half work in nursing or residential facilities, almost 30% work in hospitals, the rest work in home care

E. Work settings include
    1. Patient home
    2. Extended care facility, nursing home
    3. Assisted living/group homes
    4. Hospital palliative care or hospice inpatient unit
    5. Hospice facility
    6. Outpatient clinics
    7. Prisons
    8. Homeless shelters
    9. Adult day care centers
F. Patient populations served by hospice and palliative Nursing Assistants
    1. Infants to the elderly
    2. Patients diagnosed with life-limiting progressive diseases
G. Professional characteristics of the Nursing Assistant (also see Chapter 10)
    1. Dependable
    2. Responsible for own action
    3. Responsible to others
    4. Willing to be a team member
    5. Flexible
    6. Communicates clearly and appropriately
H. Roles of the hospice and palliative Nursing Assistant[5]
    1. Assists in meeting physical, psychosocial, spiritual, and emotional needs of patients and families experiencing life-limiting progressive illness and continuing through bereavement
        a) Physical needs: e.g., assists the patient with activities of daily living
        b) Psychosocial needs: e.g., seeks opportunities for the patient to spend time and interact with loved ones
        c) Spiritual needs: e.g., offers quiet time for prayer or reflection prior to the patient's meal
        d) Emotional needs: e.g., holds the hand of the patient when the patient is upset and listens to patient's needs
    2. Honors unique experience of each patient and family
I. In some settings, Nursing Assistants spend more time with patients and families than any other team member

> *The role of the Nursing Assistant in hospice and palliative care is to assist in meeting the physical, psychological, spiritual, and emotional needs of patients and families experiencing life-time progressive illness and continuing through bereavement.*

III. Scope of Hospice and Palliative Nursing Assistant Responsibilities

A. National Board for Certification of Hospice and Palliative Nurses (NBCHPN®) job analysis study for

1. NBCHPN® studied the role of the Nursing Assistant in caring for patients and families at the EOL

2. Study involved Nursing Assistants working in many settings, such as hospice and home care agencies, nursing homes, hospitals, and in many parts of the United States

3. Study results were used by Hospice and Palliative Nurses Association (HPNA) and NBCHPN® to develop

   a) Statement on the Scope and Standards of Hospice and Palliative Nursing Assistant Practice[5]

   b) Hospice and Palliative Nursing Assistant Competencies[6]

   c) Nursing Assistant Certification Examination

B. Scope of Practice: describes the who, what, where, when, why, and how of the specialty area of practice; describes what the practice includes and claims an area of nursing practice (such as hospice and palliative care) as a specialty[5]

C. Competencies: knowledge, attitudes, and skills the hospice and palliative Nursing Assistant demonstrates when providing quality care for seriously ill patients and their families[6]

D. Knowledge and skills required in hospice and palliative Nursing Assistant practice[5,6]

1. Physical, psychosocial, emotional, and spiritual care of patient and family experiencing life-limiting progressive illness, dying, death, and bereavement

2. Understanding of how each patient's and family's culture, values, spirituality, and experiences influence care at EOL

3. Principles of decision making and treatment goal-setting

4. Loss and grief

5. Patient education and advocacy

6. Bereavement care

7. Ethical and legal considerations in providing EOL care

8. Listening and communication skills specific to EOL care

9. Available community resources for dying patients and their families

10. Compassionate care for all individuals

11. Self awareness and ability to perform self-care

E. *Hospice and Palliative Nursing Assistant Core Curriculum* is based on the job analysis study and HPNA *Statement on the Scope and Standards of Hospice and Palliative Nursing Assistant Practice*[5]

IV. Summary

A. The major goal of hospice and palliative care is to enhance the quality of life for patients and their families facing progressive, life-limiting illnesses

B. Nursing Assistants play a central role on hospice and palliative care teams, often providing much of the hands-on care

C. Hospice and Palliative Nurses Association has developed standards of care and professional opportunities for Nursing Assistants working with patients and families at the EOL

CITED REFERENCES

1. American Association of Colleges of Nursing (AACN) and the City of Hope National Medical Center. Module I: Principles of Palliative Care. *End-of-Life Nursing Education Consortium (ELNEC) - Geriatric*; 2008.
2. Edwards M, Ersek M. Module 1: Overview of Hospice and Palliative Care. *Nursing Assistant Computerized Education Program (NA-CEP)*. Pittsburgh, PA: Hospice and Palliative Nurses Association; 2006.
3. National Consensus Project (NCP) for Quality Palliative Care. *National Consensus Project for Quality Palliative Care: Clinical Practice Guidelines for Quality Palliative Care,* 2nd ed. Pittsburgh, PA: National Consensus Project for Quality Palliative Care; 2009.
4. Bureau of Labor Statistics, U.S. Department of Labor, *Occupational Outlook Handbook, 2008-09 Edition, Nursing, Psychiatric, and Home Health Aides;* Available at: www.bls.gov/oco/ocos165.htm. Accessed October 15, 2008.
5. Hospice and Palliative Nurses Association. *Statement on the Scope and Standards of Hospice and Palliative Nursing Assistant Practice.* Pittsburgh, PA: Hospice and Palliative Nurses Association; 2009.
6. Hospice and Palliative Nurses Association. H*ospice and Palliative Nursing Assistant Competencies.* Pittsburgh, PA: Hospice and Palliative Nurses Association; 2009.

ADDITIONAL REFERENCES AND RESOURCES

Ferrell BR, Coyle N, eds. *Textbook of Palliative Nursing,* 2nd ed. New York, NY: Oxford University Press; 2006.

CHAPTER 2
PAIN MANAGEMENT AT THE END OF LIFE

Kimberly M. Bergen, MSN RN

Original Author
Jayne Pawasauskas, PharmD

I. **Pain: Definition, Prevalence at the End of Life, and Types of Pain**
   A. Pain is a human experience
      1. Pain is more than the nerve signals that result from tissue injury or physical damage
      2. Patient's emotional, social, spiritual, and physical response is a central part of the experience
         a) Explains how two patients having a similar injury may react very differently
         b) No predictable relationship between amount or size of the injury and the feeling of pain
      3. Because pain is an experience, another useful definition is that "pain is whatever the person experiencing it says it is"[1]

   > *Pain is what the patient says it is!*
   > *M. McCaffery*

   B. *Myths* about pain
      1. It is normal to have pain as you get older
      2. If you are older or have dementia, you are less sensitive to pain
      3. If you do not report pain, you probably are not having any
      4. If you can sleep at night, you do not really have pain
      5. If you use pain medications, you will get addicted to them
   C. Pain is a common symptom at the end of life
      1. 65-80% of patients with terminal cancer have pain[2]
      2. 71-83% of nursing home residents experience pain[3]
      3. 25-50% of community-dwelling elderly have pain that interferes with their daily activities[3]
   D. Types of pain
      1. Acute and chronic pain (see Table 1)
      2. Nociceptive pain
         a) Pain that comes from
            i. Tissues, such as bones, joints, skin, muscles
            ii. Organs, such as stomach, intestines, heart
         b) Examples
            i. Sprained ankle or broken bone
            ii. Gall stones

	ACUTE PAIN	**CHRONIC PAIN**
TABLE 1. Differences Between Acute and Chronic Pain		
Onset	Sudden	Gradual or sudden
Duration	Less than three months or as long as it takes for the normal healing process to occur	Longer than three months; chronic pain may start from an acute injury or event but continues past the time expected for healing to occur
Severity	Mild to severe	Mild to severe
Cause of the pain	Generally, one can identify a triggering event or illness (e.g., injury, surgery)	May not be known, and original cause of the pain may differ from the mechanisms that maintain the chronic pain
Course of the pain	Decreases over time and goes away on its own as healing occurs	Typically, the pain does not go away, although there may be periods when it improves -- waxing and waning pattern
Typical physical and behavioral signs and symptoms	Flight or fight (stress) response: • ↑ heart rate • ↑ respiratory rate • ↑ blood pressure • Sweating, pale skin • Anxiety, agitation, confusion	Usually chronic pain has behavioral signs and symptoms: • Little emotional expression or response (flat affect) • Decreased physical movement/activity • Feeling tired, fatigued • Decreased social interaction
Usual goals of treatment	Pain control with eventual elimination of the pain	Pain control to the extent possible; focus on enhancing function and quality of life

       iii.   Muscle aches

       iv.   Arthritis

   c)   Pain from tissues, such as muscles, is usually described as dull or aching

   d)   Pain from organs is usually described as deep, squeezing, or crampy

3.   Neuropathic pain (nerve pain)

   a)   Pain that results from injury to the nerves or central nervous system (central nervous system = spinal cord and brain)

   b)   Examples

       i.   Pain from shingles (also called postherpetic neuralgia)

       ii.   Pain in the hands and feet from diabetes

       iii.   Pain following a stroke

   c)   Often described as burning, stabbing, or radiating pain

4.   Referred pain

   a)   Pain that is felt in a part of the body away from the area where the pain starts

    b) Examples
        i. Heart pain (angina) can be felt in the jaw, ear, back, or arm (most often left side)
        ii. Gallbladder pain may be felt in the shoulder area
        iii. Liver pain may be felt in neck or mid-back
  E. Psychosocial pain, spiritual pain, and suffering (also see Chapters 7 and 8)
     1. Pain that comes from sadness and loss
     2. Pain that cannot be relieved with medication
  F. Pain management involves entire team, including Nursing Assistants, physical therapists, social workers, chaplains, and other spiritual counselors

II. Pain Observation and Reporting

  A. Pain is the fifth vital sign; observe the patient often for pain and report it right away

  B. When to observe the patient and ask about pain

> *Pain is the 5th vital sign.*

     1. Before and during personal care
     2. Before, during, and after transfers and ambulation
     3. Before and after activities
     4. At appropriate times after pain management therapies
        a) Talk with the nurse or other team members about the best time to observe pain after specific medications are given
        b) For example, observe or ask patients about 20 minutes after they receive fast-acting morphine—that is when it should begin to work; the peak effect for this medication should be observed about 60 minutes after it is given
     5. Whenever patient reports pain or you observe pain
  C. Believe the patient's report of pain
  D. Information from people who spend a lot of time with the patient (family, friends, etc.) is valuable because pain may show up as small changes in patient's behavior
  E. Pain may have a different meaning to different patients
  F. Patients sometimes will use different words to describe their pain, such as achiness, soreness, or discomfort
  G. Several pain assessment tools exist, but the basic information is similar
  H. Elements of pain observation
     1. Location: Where is the pain? Make sure to get information about all the places the patient has pain
     2. Severity or intensity: how bad is the pain?
        a) Important to ask how bad the pain is because mild (rating of 1-3 on a 0-10 scale), moderate (4-6 on a scale of 10) or severe (7-10 on a scale of 0-10) often need different types and dosages of pain medicine
        b) Examples of pain intensity scales
           i. Numerical rating scale (Figure 1)
              (a) Ask: "If zero is no pain and ten is the worst possible pain you can imagine, what is your pain right now?"
              (b) Ask what is the worst and the least that the pain has been in the past week

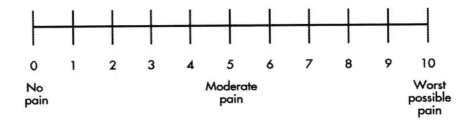

Figure 1: Numerical Rating Scale (NRS)
May be duplicated for use in clinical practice. As appears in McCaffery M, Pasero C. Pain: Clinical manual, p.67, 1999, Mosby, Inc.

  ii. Wong-Baker FACES Scale (Figure 2)
    (a) Use with children
    (b) Ask the patient to tell you which face best describes how he or she is feeling about the pain

Figure 2: Wong-Baker FACES Pain Rating Scale
Modified from Wong DL: Whaley and Wong's Essentials of Pediatric Nursing. 5th ed. St. Louis, MO: Mosby;1997:1215-1216.

  iii. Verbal descriptor scale
    (a) Patient chooses word or phrase that best describes pain
    (b) No pain – mild pain – discomforting – distressing – intense – excruciating
    (c) No pain – mild pain – moderate pain – severe pain – very severe pain – worst possible pain
  iv. Adult FACES scale (Figure 3)
    (a) Instructions: Show the patient the scale and ask: "This face (point to Face #1) shows someone with no pain. These faces show more and more pain (point to each from left to right) up to this one (point to Face #7) shows the worst pain possible. Point to the face that shows how much you hurt [right now]."
  v. Pain thermometer (Figure 4)
 c) Use large-type visual scales whenever possible
 d) The team will try different scales until the patient finds one that is easy for him/her to understand and use, then use the same scale every time
3. Timing – when does it hurt?
 a) Is your pain always there? In other words, is it constant?
 b) Does your pain come and go? In other words, is it intermittent?

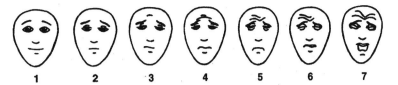

Figure 3: Adult FACES Pain Scale

Adapted from Pain 1990;41(2):139-150. NL,

Used with permission from Elsevier Science – NL, Sara Biergerjartstraat 25. 1055 KV Amsterdam, The Netherlands.

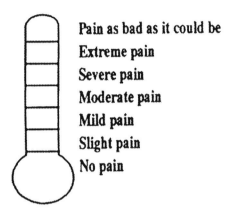

Figure 4: Pain Thermometer

From Herr K. Assessment of Persistent Pain. *JAGS* 2002;50(6): 3-7.

4. Quality of the pain: ask patient to describe the pain
   a) Crushing
   b) Dull
   c) Aching
   d) Stabbing
   e) Pinching
   f) Sharp
   g) Gnawing
   h) Pressure
5. What makes the pain worse?
   a) Moving around
   b) Fatigue
   c) Lying still
6. What makes the pain better?
   a) Medicines
   b) Social activities
   c) Non-drug therapies such as massage, distraction
7. How does the pain affect the patient?
   a) Does the pain make it hard for the patient to sleep?
   b) Does the pain affect the patient's appetite?

    c) Does the pain make it hard for the patient to move around or do physical activities?

    d) Does the pain get in the way of the patient's ability to interact with other people?

    e) Does the pain make the patient feel sad, frightened, angry, anxious?

    f) Does the pain make it hard for the patient to think clearly?

8. Are there cultural, spiritual, or personal aspects of the patient's expression of pain? (see Chapters 6 and 8)

9. Is the patient experiencing any side effects of pain medications such as drowsiness, nausea, or constipation?

10. Pain in patients who are unable to talk or report their pain[4]

    a) Many patients we care for are unable to express their pain to us in words; these patients include

        i. Infants and very young children

        ii. Patients who are in a coma

        iii. Patients with advanced dementia

        iv. Patients with severe developmental disabilities

        v. Patients who are confused or delirious

        vi. Patients who are very close to death

        vii. Patients with certain brain disorders

    b) For these patients, we need to look at behaviors to see if they are in pain. These behaviors include

        i. Sounds: moans, grunts, sighing

        ii. Facial expressions: grimacing, wincing, frowning, clenched teeth

        iii. Breathing: noisy and labored

        iv. Body movements: restlessness, rocking, pacing

        v. Body tension: clenched fist, stiff arms and legs

        vi. Resisting care: pushing people away, hitting, or scratching others

    c) There are also special tools for observing pain in non-verbal patients, such as

        i. The FLACC (Face-Legs-Activity-Cry-Consolability)[6]; use with infants and young children (see Table 2)

    d) Always promptly report behaviors that may indicate the patient is in pain or uncomfortable

    e) If a person on pain medicines becomes unable to report pain, do not assume they have no pain; continue to look for pain behaviors

        i. Pain in Advanced Dementia (PAIN-AD)[7] (See Table 3)

III. Managing Pain at the End of Life

    A. General Nursing Assistant actions to help manage the patient's pain

      1. Observe and report the presence and characteristics of pain

      2. Observe and report side effects of medications

      3. Observe and report the effectiveness of therapies

      4. Deliver some non-drug therapies as appropriate

      5. Communicate patient and family goals for pain relief to other team members

      6. Provide emotional and physical comfort to patients and families

Category	Scoring		
	1	**2**	**3**
Face	No particular expression or smile	Occasional grimace or frown, withdrawn, disinterested	Frequent to constant quivering chin, clenched jaw
Legs	Normal position or relaxed	Uneasy, restless, tense	Kicking, or legs drawn up
Activity	Lying quietly, normal position, moves easily	Squirming, shifting back and forth, tense	Arched, rigid or jerking
Cry	No cry (awake or sleep)	Moans or whimpers; occasional complaint	Crying steadily, screams or sobs, frequent complaints
Consolability	Content, relaxed	Reassured by occasional touching, hugging or being talked to, distractible	Difficult to console or comfort

Table 2: FLACC Scale

Each of the five categories (F) Face; (L) Legs; (A) Activity; (C) Cry; (C) Consolability is scored from 0-2, which results in a total score between zero and ten.

From Merkel S, et al. *The FLACC: a behavioral scale for scoring postoperative pain in young children.* Pediatric Nurse. 1997;23(3):293-297. Copyright 1997 by Jannetti Co. University of Michigan Medical Center. Reprinted with permission.

	0	1	2	Score
Breathing Independent of vocalization	Normal	Occasional labored breathing. Short period of hyperventilation	Noisy labored breathing. Long period of hyperventilation. Cheyne-stokes respirations	
Negative Vocalization	None	Occasional moan or groan. Low level speech with a negative or disapproving quality	Repeated troubled calling out. Loud moaning or groaning. Crying	
Facial expression	Smiling, or inexpressive	Sad. Frightened. Frown	Facial grimacing	
Body Language	Relaxed	Tense. Distressed pacing. Fidgeting	Rigid. Fists clenched, Knees pulled up. Pulling or pushing away. Striking out	
Consolability	No need to console	Distracted or reassured by voice or touch	Unable to console, Distract or reassure	
			TOTAL	

Table 3: Pain Assessment IN Advanced Dementia – PAINAD (Warden, Hurley, Volicer, 2003)

B. Managing pain is important because uncontrolled pain can cause other problems such as
 1. Decreased quality of life
 2. Changes in sleep patterns
 3. Changes in appetite
 4. Changes in level of functioning
 5. Increased risk for becoming depressed
C. Medicines for pain (analgesics)
 1. Pain medicines generally are used in a stepwise approach, beginning with a medicine such as acetaminophen (Tylenol®) for mild pain and using a narcotic (opioid) such as morphine for moderate or severe pain
 2. Using more than one type of pain medicine often is helpful; be sure you know all the pain medicines your patient is on so you can observe for side effects
 3. Many ways to give pain medicines (morphine in particular, can be administered by most routes)
  a) By mouth (oral)
  b) Rectally
  c) Into the skin (subcutaneous)
  d) Under the tongue (sublingual)
  e) Through the vein (intravenous)
  f) Through skin (transdermal)
  g) Through the spine (epidural, intraspinal)
 4. Types of pain medicines
  a) Acetaminophen (Tylenol®)
   i. Usually tried before other pain medicines, especially in mildly or moderately painful conditions
   ii. Often combined with other medications (e.g., Percocet® is a combination of oxycodone, an opioid, and acetaminophen)
   iii. Few side effects, but can cause liver damage at high doses
   iv. Wait at least 30-60 minutes after a dose is given to observe or ask patient whether or not it is effective
  b) NSAIDs (non-steroidal anti-inflammatory drugs)
   i. Examples of commonly used NSAIDs: ibuprofen (Motrin®, Advil®) and naproxen (Aleve®)
   ii. Can be used for fever, pain, or inflammation
   iii. Serious side effects
   iv. Bleeding problems: observe patient for signs of bleeding, e.g., vomiting of blood or coffee-ground looking material, blood in stool or dark stool
   v. Stomach upset or ulcers
   vi. Side effects are more common and more serious in elderly patients
D. Opioids
 1. Sometimes called "narcotics;" the better term is "opioids"

2. Examples
   a) Codeine (Tylenol® No. 3)
   b) Morphine (MS Contin®, Oramorph®)
   c) Oxycodone (Percocet®, OxyContin®)
   d) Hydrocodone (Vicodin®, Hycodan®)
   e) Hydromorphone (Dilaudid®)
   f) Fentanyl (Duragesic®) "the pain patch"
   g) Methadone (Dolophine®)

3. Duration of action
   a) Short-acting: often used as needed (prn) for intermittent pain or for patients who have just started on opioids
   b) Long-acting: more useful and appropriate for chronic, constant pain

4. Common side effects of opioids
   a) Drowsiness: usually happens at start of treatment or when dose is increased and improves after a few days. Monitor patient for falls
   b) Respiratory depression: defined as breathing less than 8 times per minute in a patient who is difficult to wake up. Usually a problem only at the start of treatment or with a major dose increase
   c) Constipation: constipation occurs in most patients taking opioids; unlike nausea and sedation, constipation does not go away. Most patients start taking medications to prevent constipation. It is also helpful to encourage intake of fluids, encourage intake of fiber (e.g., fruits, and vegetables), encourage physical activity. (see Chapter 3)
   d) Nausea and vomiting: may occur at start of treatment, but usually improves after a few days. (see Chapter 3)
   e) Muscle twitching: usually occurs at higher doses
   f) Pruritus (itching): most common side effect when opioids are given into the spine. Itching may be treated with other drugs such as diphenhydramine (Benadryl®)

E. Additional medications used for pain
   1. Also called co-analgesics or adjuvants
   2. Antidepressants: Used for nerve pain. Examples include nortriptyline (Pamelor®), amitriptyline (Elavil®), and desipramine (Norpramin®). Side effects include dry mouth, difficulty urinating, and drowsiness
   3. Anti-seizure medications: Used for nerve pain. Examples include carbamazepine (Tegretol®) and gabapentin (Neurontin®). Most common side effect is drowsiness
   4. Anesthetic creams, gels, sprays and patches: Example: lidocaine (Lidoderm®)
   5. Corticosteroids: Examples prednisone, dexamethasone (Decadron®)
      a) Short-term side effects can include high blood pressure, increased blood sugar, increased risk for infection, and mood changes. Long-term side effects include swelling, fragile skin, and bone weakness

F. Non-drug pain management strategies
   1. Examples of non-drug strategies
      a) Distraction/relaxation
      b) Heat/cold application

        c)   Massage

        d)   Imagery

        e)   Controlled breathing

        f)   Music

        g)   Comfort foods

        h)   Exercise

        i)   Positioning

2. Best used along with medicines; e.g., play relaxing music for a patient while waiting for a pain medication to take effect

3. Ask about what the patient has tried in the past and what works

4. Include family or caregiver, when possible; teach family or caregiver how to provide these therapies

5. Talk with the nurse about which non-drug therapies to use and whether there are special issues to consider; e.g., a patient with severe bone cancer should not be massaged

        a)   Instructions for specific strategies

        b)   Distraction: collect several pictures. Ask the patient to look at one picture and describe what he or she sees. Have the patient talk about the picture or imagine being in the picture or ask the patient to make up a story about the picture. Teach the family or caregiver how to do this, or have them bring some old photographs to use for this strategy

        c)   Relaxation, deep breathing exercise: speak to the patient slowly and say "Breath in slowly and deeply. As you breathe out, feel your self begin to relax. Now, breathe in and out slowly and regularly. Imagine doing this in a place that is relaxing for you." Repeat these steps for up to 20 minutes. End with a slow, deep breath, and ask the patient to say or think, "I feel alert and relaxed."

        d)   Massage: Examples: Brief touch, such as hand holding or rubbing someone's shoulder, giving a gentle foot or hand massage

IV. Barriers to Effective Pain Management

A. Although there are many effective therapies for pain, patients still have unrelieved pain at the end of life

B. Major barriers

1. Healthcare providers

        a)   Lack of knowledge about pain management

        b)   Poor pain observation and assessment

        c)   Concerns about addiction and tolerance

        d)   Concern about side effects

2. Patients and families

        a)   Reluctance to report pain, not wanting to "complain"

        b)   Concern about distracting the physician from treating the disease

        c)   Fear of addiction and tolerance to pain medications

        d)   Concern about side effects

C. Nursing assistants must have accurate knowledge about pain management to calm their own fears and to give support to patients and families[5]

   1. Fear of addiction

      a) Many patients and families are afraid that taking opioids will make the patients addicted. Nursing Assistants need to know what addiction is and what it is not

      b) Opioid addiction is a chronic disease in which people have poor control over drug use, and use a drug for reasons other than pain, e.g., using the drug to get high. They crave the drug and use it even though it causes serious physical or social problems

      c) Addiction is uncommon in people with pain at end of life

      d) Fear of addiction is not a good reason to discourage the use of opioids to manage pain

      e) If you are worried that the patient might be addicted to the pain medicine, talk with the nurse

   2. Tolerance

      a) Tolerance to pain medicine happens when patients use the medicine for weeks or months and find that they need higher doses over time to get good pain relief; it is like their body "gets used to the drug" and needs more to keep the same effects

      b) Usually, a need to increase the dose is the result of the disease getting worse rather than the patient developing tolerance to the drug

      c) Some patients are afraid that if they take strong painkillers early in the illness, they will not work later on. This is not true, although tolerance can occur

      d) When tolerance does occur, the dose can be increased so the patient gets good relief

      e) Tolerance does not mean the patient is addicted

   3. Physical dependence

      a) When patients are physically dependent on a drug, they go through withdrawal if the medication is stopped or decreased quickly

      b) Withdrawal happens with opioids, as well as other medications

      c) _Any_ person who is on regular doses of opioids for weeks or months will become physically dependent

      d) Physical dependence does not mean the patient is addicted

V. Summary

A. Pain is one of the most common and most distressing symptoms at the end of life

B. Successful pain control needs involvement of the entire team, including the family

C. Important Nursing Assistant roles include

   1. Observing for pain and reporting it promptly

   2. Observing for side effects of pain medications

   3. Administering some non-drug therapies, especially helping the patient to focus on something other than pain

   4. Providing emotional support to patients and families

CITED REFERENCES

1. McCaffery M, Pasero C. *Pain: Clinical manual.* 2nd ed. St. Louis, MO: Mosby; 1999.
2. American Pain Society. *Pain: Current Understanding of Assessment, Management and Treatments.* 2006.
3. American Geriatrics Society. The management of persistent pain in older persons. *Journal of the American Geriatrics Society* 2002;50 Suppl 6:1-20.
4. Herr K, Coyne PJ, Key T, Manworren R, McCaffery M, Merkel S, Pelosi-Kelly J, Wild L, et al. Pain assessment in the nonverbal patient: position statement with clinical practice recommendations. *Pain Management Nursing.* 2006;7:44-52.
5. Zeigler DG, Howell HR. Opioid addiction: no reason to withhold pain management. *US Pharmacist 2008.* Available at: www.uspharmacist.com/index.asp?page=ce/105745/default.htm. Accessed September 24, 2008.
6. Merkel SI, Voepel-Lewis T, Shayevitz JR, Malviya S. The FLACC: a behavioral scale for scoring postoperative pain in young children. *Pediatric Nursing.* 1997;23(3):293-297.
7. Warden V, Hurley AC, Volicer L. Development and psychometric evaluation of the Pain Assessment in Advanced Dementia (PAINAD) Scale. *Journal of the American Medical Directors.* 2003;4(1):9-15.

ADDITIONAL REFERENCES AND RESOURCES

American Association of Colleges of Nursing and the City of Hope National Medical Center. Module 2: Pain management. *End-of-Life Nursing Education Consortium (ELNEC) - Geriatric,* 2008.

Ersek M, ed. *Nursing Assistant End-of-life Care Computerized Education Program (NA-CEP).* Pittsburgh, PA: Hospice and Palliative Nurses Association; 2006.

Resources available at www.hpna.org

HPNA Patient/Family Teaching Sheets

❖ *Managing Pain*
❖ *Managing Opioid Induced Constipation*

HPNA TIPs Sheets

❖ *TIPs for Dispelling Myths of Opioids*
❖ *TIPs for Managing Opioid Induced Constipation*
❖ *TIPs for Recognizing Behaviors Indicating Patient Has Pain*
❖ *TIPs for Recognizing Pain in Patients with the Inability to Communicate Verbally*
❖ *TIPs for the Nursing Assistant Role in Pain Management*

HPNA Position Statement

❖ *Pain Management*

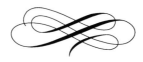

CHAPTER 3
MANAGEMENT OF OTHER SYMPTOMS AT THE END OF LIFE

Patricia Berry, PhD, APRN, GNP-BC, ACHPN®

Original Author
Beth Miller Kraybill, RN, BSN, CHPN®

I. **Introduction**
  A. Definitions
    1. Signs: objective indicators of illness; things that can be seen by an observer; e.g., fever as a sign of infection; lack of urine as a sign of kidney failure; increased respiratory rate as a sign of difficulty breathing
    2. Symptoms: subjective features of illness as defined by the person experiencing them; e.g., pain and nausea; descriptions of symptoms often include
      a) Frequency (how often the symptom occurs)
      b) Duration (how long the symptom lasts)
      c) Amount of distress experienced by the person
  B. Why is the management of symptoms important?
    1. Unrelieved symptoms
      a) Interfere with activities of daily living (ADLs), e.g., walking, eating sleeping, taking care of oneself
      b) Cause distress and suffering
      c) Decrease quality of life (QOL)
    2. Managing symptoms quickly may prevent a negative cycle: increased discomfort → distress, including anxiety → more discomfort → suffering
  C. Frequency of symptoms
    1. People with progressive, life-limiting illness often experience many symptoms
    2. Rather than reviewing all end-of-life (EOL) symptoms, this chapter will focus on nine of the most commonly occurring symptoms
  D. Nursing Assistant roles in symptom management
    1. Observation and reporting
      a) The Nursing Assistant often spends more time with patients and families than other team members, so they are best able to observe, interact with the patient and family and collect information
      b) Information about symptoms can be collected by
        i. Observing and listening for signs (e.g., wet or noisy breathing, red or open areas on the skin) and symptoms (e.g., patient tells you they "feel shaky" when they get out of the bed or a chair)
        ii. Watching for signs (e.g., agitation, confusion, restlessness)

> *Symptom Management is important for quality of life.*

iii. Measuring blood pressure, pulse, respiratory rate, temperature, urine output

iv. Talking with the patient, family or other caregivers (e.g. staff in assisted living or nursing home, volunteers)

2. Working with other team members, reporting symptoms and signs, helping manage symptoms under the direction of the nurse; observing and reporting side effects of medicines used to manage symptoms

3. Providing emotional support to patient and family

II. Common Symptoms

A. Anorexia

1. Definition

a) Anorexia: lack of appetite and loss of desire to eat

b) Cachexia: "wasting," weight loss, loss of muscle mass; often occurs with weakness

c) Lack of appetite occurs throughout the course of illness and anorexia is nearly always present in advanced disease and at the end of life

2. Causes

a) Conditions such as tumors of the stomach or esophagus, depression and/or anxiety, increased pressure in the brain from tumors or stroke, mouth, and stomach infections

b) Treatment-related, e.g., medication side effects (nausea, constipation), mouth ulcers from chemotherapy, taste changes due to radiation or chemotherapy

c) Poorly fitting dentures

3. Observe and report

a) Increased weakness or inability to perform ADLs

b) Weight loss

c) Patient report of sore mouth or throat or unrelieved heartburn

d) Patient report of feeling full after eating very small amounts of food

e) No bowel movement in the past 3 or more days

f) Patient report of have difficulties with bowel movements

g) Patient report or family/caregiver observation of sad mood or depression

h) Dry mouth, chapped, or cracked lips

4. Nursing Assistant interventions

a) Identify patient's favorite foods and encourage other caregivers to offer these food often and in small servings

b) Provide high-calorie nutritious snacks, if appropriate

c) Assist with good mouth care

d) Support family members and assure them that lack of appetite is very common at EOL; anorexia is often of particular concern to the family in the following ways

i. Preparing and providing food is a central part of daily life for many families

    ii. Patient's lack of interest in food can be seen by the family as a personal rejection rather than a physical symptom

    iii. Family members often worry that the patient is "starving"

  e) Instruct patient to avoid strong or unpleasant odors; patient may need to stay away from the kitchen; room temperature or cold foods may be better tolerated than hot foods

  f) Report patient or family comments or questions about artificial feeding or hydration

  g) Especially important in the final weeks of life: offer sips of favorite liquids and ice chips; keep the patient's mouth clean and keep the lips moist with lip balm or other non-petroleum-based product

 5. Medical treatment (will depend upon the goals of care)

  a) Earlier in the disease, therapy may include: a dietary consult; monitoring of intake and weight, appetite stimulating medications, such as dexamethasone (Decadron®) or megestrol (Megace®)

  b) For patients receiving hospice care, intense dietary and weight monitoring is rarely necessary; eating for pleasure should be the goal

  c) Artificial nutrition and hydration usually are not appropriate at the EOL because they rarely help the patient to gain weight or feel better

B. Constipation

 1. Definition: varies depending on patient's normal bowel pattern; generally agreed to be bowel movements (BMs) that are infrequent (that is, less than once every three days) and difficult to pass due to hardness

 2. Causes

  a) Disease or conditions such as colon cancer, neuromuscular diseases (e.g., multiple sclerosis, amyotrophic lateral sclerosis or ALS disease [also called Lou Gehrig's]), diabetes, hemorrhoids

  b) Treatment-related causes, such as medication side effects, especially pain medicines; e.g., morphine, hydrocodone (Lortab®), oxycodone (OxyContin®; Percocet®)

  c) Other causes

    i. Decreased intake of food

    ii. Inability to maintain adequate fluid and fiber intake

    iii. Immobility or lack of exercise

    iv. Lack of privacy

    v. Generalized pain

    vi. Weakness

 3. Observe and report

  a) A change in patient's normal bowel pattern

    i. BMs less than once in 3 days

    ii. Patient report or Nursing Assistant observation of patient straining to have a BM or very hard stool, small amounts of stool

  b) Nausea and vomiting that is not related to other causes, such as a stomach virus

  c) Increased bloating

    d)   Abdominal pain or fullness

    e)   Oozing of liquid stool, which may be a sign of impaction

    f)   Increase in gas passed without BM

4. Nursing Assistant interventions

    a)   Encourage fluids as the patient can tolerate

    b)   Suggest warm drink, such as tea or water, in the morning

    c)   Provide privacy

    d)   Encourage exercise if appropriate with the goals of care

    e)   Suggest regular time of day to attempt to move bowels

    f)   Encourage patient to sit upright while trying to move bowels

    g)   Warm washcloth to rectum can be soothing if patient has rectal soreness

5. Medical treatment

    a)   Medications of many types, most often used in combination

        i.   Stool softeners: e.g., docusate sodium (DOSS®, Colace®)

        ii.   Stimulant laxatives: e.g., senna (Senokot®), bisacodyl (Dulcolax®)

        iii.   Rectal suppositoires: e.g., glycerin, bisacodyl (Dulcolax®)

        iv.   Enemas: e.g., sodium phosphate (Fleet Phospho-Soda®)

        v.   Herbal preparations: psyllium seed, flaxseed

        vi.   Methylnaltrexone (Relistor®) maybe used for opioid induced constipation not relieved by other laxatives

    b)   Manual disimpaction

C. Dyspnea

1. Definition: difficult or labored breathing; also described as extreme shortness of breath or breathlessness

    a)   Very distressing sensation: patient may fear suffocation and family caregivers may feel helpless

    b)   Different than Cheyne-Stokes breathing, which is a pattern of irregular breathing with increasing apnea (lack of breathing) that is common in the final hours or days of life; Cheyne-Stokes breathing is not usually distressing to the patient

2. Causes

    a)   Disease or infectious processes, such as

        i.   Cancer of the lung

        ii.   Congestive heart failure

        iii.   Pneumonia

        iv.   Anemia (lack of red blood cells that carry oxygen)

        v.   Pulmonary embolus (blood clot in lung)

        vi.   Ascites (fluid in the abdomen)

        vii.   Lung diseases, such as emphysema, or chronic obstructive pulmonary disease (COPD)

        viii.   Amyotrophic lateral sclerosis or ALS disease (also called Lou Gehrig's) and other neuromuscular diseases

        ix.   General weakness from being sick

b) Other causes include anxiety or fear

3. Observe and report

    a) Patient report of shortness of breath or air hunger

    b) Noisy breathing, gasping

    c) Anxious expression

    d) Flaring nostrils

    e) Exaggerated movement of the chest and abdomen

    f) Cyanosis (slight blue or gray coloring around lips, eyes, earlobes)

    g) Restlessness

4. Nursing Assistant interventions

    a) Open the window or use a fan to increase ventilation; aim fan directly at the cheek or nose if tolerated by patient

    b) Help patient sit as upright as possible

        i. Sitting in chair or at edge of bed

        ii. Raise head of bed

        iii. Use pillows for support

    c) If possible, drape patient's arms over bedside table, padding the table with a pillow

    d) Cool the room by turning the thermostat down or opening a window for fresh, cooler, air; offer cool damp cloths to the neck or forehead

    e) Keep items close to decrease need for exertion, e.g., place commode, telephone, and TV remote control near patient

    f) Provide distraction

    g) Provide emotional support to both patient and family

    h) Create a calming atmosphere using music or lowered lighting

5. Medical treatment differs according to disease process and stage of illness

    a) Medications

        i. Opioids: e.g., morphine

        ii. Anti-anxiety agents: e.g., lorazepam (Ativan®), alprazolam (Xanax®)

        iii. Bronchodilators: e.g., ipratropium (Atrovent®), albuterol (Proventil®)

        iv. Cough suppressants

        v. Antibiotics for lung infections: e.g., pneumonia

        vi. Diuretics: e.g., furosemide (Lasix®)

    b) Oxygen therapy

D. Fatigue

1. Definition: profound tiredness, which is unrelieved by rest, with lack of physical and mental energy, and weakness that interferes with ADLs

2. Most common symptom at EOL

3. Causes

    a) Disease and treatments, such as

        i. Anemia

        ii. Infection

        iii.   Malnutrition

        iv.   Chemical imbalance in the body

        v.   Medication side effects

        vi.   Radiation or chemotherapy side effects

        vii.   Unrelieved symptoms; e.g., pain, diarrhea, vomiting, straining with constipation

        viii.   Insomnia (inability to sleep)

   b)   Emotional factors

        i.   Stress and anxiety

        ii.   Depression

        iii.   Family conflict

        iv.   Spiritual distress

4.   Observation and Reporting

        i.   Patient reports feeling exhausted, having no energy, being tired or weary, feeling "wiped out"

        ii.   Patient or family reports patient has daytime sleepiness

        iii.   Increase in falls or accidental injury

        iv.   Patient is lethargic (lacks energy) or apathetic (not caring or showing enthusiasm)

5.   Nursing Assistant interventions

   a)   Encourage energy-saving techniques when assisting with ADLs, e.g., commode at bedside, toiletry items within easy reach

   b)   Help the patient focus on the activities he/she most wants to do and learn to ask others for help

   c)   Promote independence by creative arrangement of the environment

        i.   In home setting, suggest moving patient bed to main floor or close to bedroom door

        ii.   Ensure chairs or stools are available for sitting if the house or facility has long halls; place chairs in several locations in large rooms

        iii.   Encourage installation and use of grab bars or rails

   d)   Decrease risk of falls by

        i.   Removing throw rugs and obstacles in the patient's path

        ii.   Make sure patient has a hand bell or call light to call for help when needed

   e)   Encourage frequent rest periods; suggest limiting time in bed during day to improve night-time sleep

   f)   Provide emotional support to family; they may express feelings that the patient is "giving up," and may need help understanding that the patient cannot control fatigue and that it is the most common EOL symptom

   g)   Encourage patient to feel good about accomplishments and not be critical of himself or herself for inability to be active

   h)   Encourage pleasant activities that restore energy, for instance, going outdoors, listening to music, pet therapy

6. Medical treatment
   a) Medications
      i. Steroids: e.g., dexamethasone (Decadron®)
      ii. Stimulants: e.g., methylphenidate (Ritalin®), pemoline (Cylert®)
      iii. Antidepressants : e.g., (fluoxetine (Prozac®), paroxetine (Paxil®)
      iv. Erythropoietin (Epogen®) to increase red blood cell production
   b) Blood transfusions for anemia
   c) Management of other symptoms, such as nausea, pain, depression, and constipation
7. Other approaches (depending on goals of care)
   a) Mild exercise program
   b) Physical therapy
   c) Occupational therapy

E. Nausea and vomiting
   1. Definition
      a) Nausea: stomach upset, often accompanied with a feeling of need to vomit or "throw up"
      b) Vomiting: forceful expelling of stomach contents through the mouth and/or nose
   2. Causes include
      a) Diseases such as kidney failure, stomach or colon cancer
      b) Medications such as antibiotics, opioids
      c) Chemotherapy
      d) Radiation therapy to gastrointestinal tract (GI)
      e) Constipation
      f) Pain
      g) Bowel obstruction
      h) Emotional distress, anxiety
   3. Observe and report
      a) Patient's report of upset stomach or queasiness, "sick to my stomach"
      b) Inability to keep down food or fluid
      c) Lack of appetite
      d) Constipation
      e) Report of specific "triggers," such as thinking about chemotherapy, smell of fried foods
   4. Nursing Assistant interventions
      a) Emotional support and reassurance
      b) Offer frequent small meals
      c) Advise patient to avoid strong food odors
      d) Serve food and fluid at preferred temperature (cold or room temperature)
      e) Advise patient to avoid foods that cause nausea (for some people, these foods include sweet, spicy, or fatty items)
      f) Provide food with smooth textures, or liquids (e.g., ginger ale, sherbet, ice cream, or clear liquids)

g) Encourage patient to eat slowly

h) Offer frequent, thorough mouth care

i) Open windows or have fan blowing

j) Offer cool damp cloth for neck or forehead

k) Participate in distraction activities

l) Encourage use of relaxation techniques

5. Medical treatment

   a) Medications: antiemetics such as prochlorperazine (Compazine®), promethazine (Phenergan®), metoclopramide (Reglan®)

6. Multidisciplinary therapies (performed by specially trained therapists)

   a) Hypnosis

   b) Acupuncture

   c) Biofeedback

F. Noisy respirations

1. Definition: moist, noisy respirations commonly called "death rattle"

2. Cause: the pooling of oral and respiratory secretions at the back of the throat, with an inability to cough and clear airway

3. Most commonly occurs in comatose patient or as death nears

4. Often is very distressing for family to hear

5. Observe and report

   a) Noisy rattling in upper airway or chest

   b) Presence of secretions in mouth

   c) Drooling of secretions

   d) Family caregiver report of any of these symptoms

6. Nursing Assistant interventions

   a) Support the family and reassure them that the patient is not experiencing distress and is not drowning

   b) Avoid term of "death rattle" in front of family and other caregivers as it brings up strong emotions; use the words "congestion" or "noisy breathing"

   c) Help prepare family that patient is in final stages of dying

   d) Reposition to alternating sides; positioning on the left side promotes drainage and can ease the noise; use pillows and other supports to position the patient way up on his/her side with the head of the bed raised

   e) Provide and suggest to the family caregiver to perform frequent oral care

   f) Reinforce that suctioning is not usually necessary and often causes more discomfort for the patient

7. Medical treatment

   a) Medications that dry secretions; e.g., scopolamine (Transderm Scop®), atropine, hyoscyamine (Levsin® drops), glycopyrrolate (Robinul®)

   b) Gentle suctioning of the mouth only if secretions can be seen

G. Terminal restlessness/delirium
 1. Definition: excessive restlessness with increased mental and physical activity
 2. Causes: at end of life, this symptom is often caused by organ failure (e.g., liver, kidney) that causes chemical imbalances, but can also be caused or worsened by
    a) Medication side effects
    b) Dehydration
    c) Infections
    d) Hypoxia (lack of oxygen)
    e) Brain metastases (cancerous tumors that have spread to the brain)
    f) Not getting enough sleep
    g) Unresolved fears or concerns about dying
 3. Observe and report
    a) Inability to lay still
    b) Repeated attempts to get out of bed
    c) "Picking" behavior, including reaching out and grasping at the air, pulling at bedding, undressing
    d) Altered sleep patterns
    e) Hallucinations (seeing or hearing things that are not there)
    f) Garbled or confused speech
    g) Inability to communicate with others
    h) Changing levels of consciousness
    i) Family stress or exhaustion related to any of the above
 4. Nursing Assistant interventions
    a) Provide emotional support to patient
    b) Identify yourself before touching patient or performing an activity
    c) Make sure the patient is safe, e.g., pad area around bed with blankets or pillows, consider moving the mattress to the floor
    d) Avoid correcting or arguing with the patient
    e) Avoid continually reorienting patient because at this stage, patient is probably unable to be oriented and frequent attempts may increase agitation
    f) Support and teach family
       i. Acknowledge sadness of "losing contact" with their family member and the feelings of helplessness
       ii. Encourage gentle touch or massage if the patient tolerates
       iii. Encourage rest periods and time away from bedside if possible
    g) Remove unnecessary items within patient reach that could be thrown or broken
    h) Decrease environmental stimuli: turn down bright lights, turn off television, try playing calming music, avoid having many people talking at the bedside
    i) Attempt gentle hand or foot massage
 5. Medical treatment
    a) Medications: haloperidol (Haldol®), olanzapine (Zyprexa®), lorazepam (Ativan®), diazepam (Valium®)
    b) Identify and treat causes of delirium such as severe pain

H. Anxiety
   1. Definition: A feeling of apprehension, worry, uneasiness, or dread, especially about the future, often without a known specific cause; person may also describe fear
   2. Causes
      a) Uncontrolled symptoms
      b) Medication side effects
      c) Fear of the unknown
      d) Financial concerns
      e) Family conflicts
      f) Spiritual distress
   3. Observe and report
      a) Patient report of feeling anxious, worried, or "going crazy"
      b) Increased restlessness, inability to find a comfortable position
      c) Increased respiratory rate, dyspnea, decreased oxygen saturation
      d) Patient reports feeling that "heart is pounding", shaky, sweaty
      e) Ask whether there are family or spiritual concerns and whether patient would like to speak to a social worker or chaplain
   4. Nursing Assistant interventions
      a) Listen with empathy (listen for clues to the cause, such as spiritual distress)
      b) Provide reassurance
      c) Turn lights down, turn off TV, remove patient from crowded or loud areas
      d) Distract the patient, e.g., by taking the patient for a walk, playing a card game, reading aloud to the patient, turning on the TV or music
   5. Medical treatments
      a) Medications: alprazolam (Xanax®), lorazepam (Ativan®), paroxetine (Paxil®), venlafaxine (Effexor®)
      b) Management of other symptoms, e.g., pain, nausea
   6. Multidisciplinary approaches (performed by specially trained therapists, chaplain, social worker)
      a) Counseling alone or with family members
      b) Social work assistance to "put affairs in order"
      c) Guided imagery
      d) Hypnosis
      e) Progressive relaxation techniques
      f) Spiritual care
I. Depression
   1. Definition: extreme and ongoing feelings that may include sadness, hopelessness, helplessness, lack of self-worth, anger
   2. These feelings may occur normally during the dying process, but if they are severe, they should be treated
   3. Causes
      a) Disease

          i.   Diabetes

          ii.   Thyroid disease

          iii.   Dementia

          iv.   Alcoholism

          v.   Brain metastases

    b) Medication side effects or withdrawal

    c) Uncontrolled symptoms, such as pain or nausea

    d) Emotional issue

          i.   Loss of control or independence

          ii.   Fear

          iii.   Spiritual distress

          iv.   Family conflict or lack of support

4. Observe and report

    a) Patient report of feeling worthless, hopeless, "no reason to keep going"

    b) Patient reports thoughts of wanting to hurt or kill self or others

    c) Patient has frequent periods of crying

    d) Patient interacts very little with family and other caregivers

    e) Changes in appetite, energy level, sleep pattern (inability to sleep is common)

5. Nursing Assistant interventions

    a) Use active listening

    b) Avoid trying to "cheer" patient; maintain normal level of social conversation

    c) Encourage as much independence and control as possible, particularly in ADLs

    d) Provide opportunity for talking about and remembering significant events from the past

    e) Encourage use of previous helpful coping mechanisms; e.g., prayer, visits from grandchildren

    f) Provide support to family

          i.   Listen to their concerns

          ii.   Encourage participation in providing care to decrease their feelings of helplessness

          iii.   Encourage breaks from caregiving by use of volunteers or supportive friends

6. Medical treatment

    a) Medications: amitriptyline (Elavil®), sertraline (Zoloft®), paroxetine (Paxil®)

    b) Control other symptoms

7. Multidisciplinary approaches (performed by specially trained therapists, chaplain, social worker)

    a) Therapeutic counseling

    b) Spiritual care

    c) Anticipatory grief counseling for family members

    d) Guided imagery

    e) Progressive relaxation techniques

    f) Massage

IV. Summary

A. End-of-life symptom management is a challenge that requires the commitment of all care providers

B. Nursing Assistants have an important role in observing, reporting, and intervening on behalf of their patients

C. Effective prevention and treatment of symptoms enhances quality of life and eases the dying process for patients and their families

ADDITIONAL REFERENCES AND RESOURCES

1. American Association of College of Nursing (AACN) and the City of Hope National Medical Center. Module 3: Nonpain symptoms at end of life. *End-of-Life Nursing Education Consortium (ELNEC) – Geriatric;* 2008.

2. Edwards M, Ersek M. *Nursing Assistant End-of-Life Care Computerized Education Program (NA-CEP).* Pittsburgh, PA: Hospice and Palliative Nurses Association; 2006.

Resources available at www.hpna.org

HPNA Patient/Family Teaching Sheets

❖ *Final Days*
❖ *Food and Fluid at End of Life*
❖ *Managing Constipation*
❖ *Managing Shortness of Breath*
❖ *Managing Fatigue*
❖ *Assisting Families to Manage Fatigue*
❖ *Managing Nausea and Vomiting*
❖ *Managing Restlessness*
❖ *Managing Delirium*
❖ *Managing Anxiety*
❖ *Managing Depression*

HPNA TIPs Sheets

❖ *TIPs for Constipation*
❖ *TIPs for Managing Fatigue*

HPNA Quick Information Sheet

❖ *Delirium in Hospice and Palliative Patients*

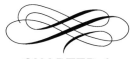

CHAPTER 4
ETHICAL ISSUES AT THE END OF LIFE

Eileen R. Chichin, PhD, RN

Original Author
Eileen R. Chichin, PhD, RN

I. **Introduction/Definition of Ethics**

A. Ethics

1. Rules or principles for doing good

2. Something we should think about in everything we do

3. When ethics involves issues in healthcare, it is often referred to as *bio*ethics ("bio" is from a Greek word, *bios,* meaning "life")

4. Especially important when you are caring for people who cannot care for themselves; e.g., infants and children or frail or sick people of any age

B. Difference between morality and ethics

1. Morality refers to what most people think is acceptable behavior

2. Ethics is the field of study that looks at what most people think is acceptable behavior (that is, what is moral) and also how society decides what is moral or immoral

C. It is important that Nursing Assistants know about ethics because they are the ones who provide most of the hands-on care to dependent people and form very close emotional attachments to them[1]

D. Definitions of some of the main ethical principles used in healthcare[2]

1. A principle is a basic idea or way of thinking that can guide us in deciding whether a particular action is right or wrong

2. Four major principles that we use in healthcare

   a) Nonmaleficence: not doing anything that is bad; first, do no harm; we are required to protect our patients from anything bad

   b) Beneficence: doing good; helping patients

   c) Autonomy: the idea that patients are allowed to make their own decisions

   > *Four major ethical principles:*
   > - *Nonmaleficence*
   > - *Beneficence*
   > - *Autonomy*
   > - *Justice*

      i. In healthcare settings, this often means that we must accept and support a decision that the patient makes, even if we ourselves might not think that is the best decision

      ii. Common examples are when a doctor suggests that a patient continue to have chemotherapy but the patient refuses, saying he has had enough; or when the healthcare team thinks the patient should have a surgical operation but the patient refuses. To respect autonomy, members of the healthcare team will go along with and support the patients' decisions although they do not agree with them

    iii. An important way in which we respect autonomy is getting informed consent from patients before giving them a treatment or doing anything to them. This means they need to be able to understand what we are telling them about the treatment, that we have to give them all the information about it, and that they agree to it without being forced to agree

  d) Justice: in healthcare settings, there are two kinds of justice

    i. Justice can mean respecting the moral or legal rights of a person, e.g., keeping something confidential

    ii. Justice also refers to how we provide care to all people who need care when there is not enough money or equipment to give care to everyone. Examples of this include not giving a heart transplant to an older person, but giving one to a younger person, or cases where doctors decide about which patient should get the last bed in an intensive care unit when several people may need intensive care

II. Ethical Dilemmas

  A. An ethical dilemma is a problem that happens because

    1. Some people believe that something may be morally right, while others believe it is morally wrong (e.g., abortion)

    2. A person believes that, on moral grounds, he or she should not do something (e.g., not give a particular medicine to keep a dying person comfortable because the medicine may make the person die sooner)

    3. Ethical dilemmas often have no "right" answer. Sometimes these dilemmas make people feel they are going against their own values. Nursing assistants should not deal with these issues alone, instead they have input as team members and should ask others for advice when they feel uncomfortable about ethical issues

    4. There are certain steps we can take to deal with ethical dilemmas and make the best decision possible. The steps include[3]

      a) Getting all the information that we can about the situation. For example, we need to know everything about the patient's physical condition and illness. Will a particular treatment cure the illness or make the person more comfortable? Will it make the person more uncomfortable? Will it make the person live longer, or die sooner? What are the pros and cons of the treatment?

      b) Use ethical principles to make the decision, e.g.,

        i. Beneficence: what would be good for the patient?

        ii. Autonomy: try to find out what the patient would want. If you do not know and the patient is unable to tell you for some reason, what do you think he would want? Why do you feel that way? Does the patient have a living will? Did he or she ask someone else to make decisions for him/her? Did he ever talk about what he would want when his condition got worse?

      c) If the team and family do not know what the patient wants, everyone should look at the benefits of the treatment (that is, what good would come from it) and the burdens of the treatment (what might be painful or uncomfortable if the treatment were given). If the burdens are greater than the benefits it may be a good idea to avoid using the treatment

   d) The team puts all the information together, that is, the patient's physical condition, his or her wishes (if they are known), the burdens and benefits of the treatment, and what is in the patient's best interest and then

      i. Works with the patient and family to make the best decision possible using all that information

      ii. Remembers that not everyone will be happy with whatever decision is made. The family may want to try to keep the patient "going" no matter what it takes, and the patient may choose to stop a particular treatment because it is too uncomfortable

III. The Relationship between What Is Legal and What Is Ethical

   A. Some things that are legal, such as capital punishment (putting someone to death for committing a very serious crime) is considered unethical by many people

   B. Other things that are illegal, such as euthanasia may be seen as ethical for some people

   C. When you work in a healthcare setting, you need to know what is legal so you can do your job properly

   D. You also need to understand that you may believe that some things are wrong (or unethical) even though they are legal. That is, just because your beliefs make you feel something is wrong does not necessarily make it wrong in the eyes of the law

IV. Everyday Ethical Issues

   A. Many times people think that ethical issues in healthcare are only things like deciding not to do cardiopulmonary resuscitation (CPR) or deciding who should get a liver transplant. However, many ethical issues are part of daily patient care

      1. An example is

         a) Giving patients choices about the time they are awakened, what clothes they wear, what they eat or drink, and whom they wish to see

      2. These everyday kinds of things are ethical issues because they are related to autonomy, beneficence, nonmaleficence, and justice

      3. We are respecting autonomy when we ask patients what they would like to wear, rather than choosing their clothing ourselves; or, not forcing patients to eat or drink when they say they do not want to

V. Common Ethical Issues at the End of Life[2,3]

   A. Who should make decisions for a patient who is too confused, or in a coma, and cannot make decisions for himself? Who should make decisions for an infant or a young child? How should medical decisions be made for a dying teenager who is able to speak for herself?

   B. How much should a patient be told about his or her medical condition?

   C. It is ethical to not give patients treatment that can save their lives?

   D. Is it ethical to not use a treatment such as a tube feeding when a patient cannot eat by mouth?

E.   Is it ethical to give very high doses of morphine for severe pain if that is the only way to keep a person comfortable even if doing so may make a person die sooner?

F.   Is it ethical to help someone commit suicide?

VI. Trends and Events that Have Influenced Bioethics and End-of-Life Care[4]

A.   Many medical technologies, e.g., CPR, feeding tubes, and kidney machines (hemodialysis), were developed in the middle of the 20th century. These technologies gave us the ability to keep people with serious illnesses alive for a long time. However, after seeing that being kept alive on machines can cause more suffering, some people felt they would not want to be kept alive with these technologies

B.   During the consumer movement of the 1970's, more patients wanted influence in making healthcare decisions that affected their lives. Before this time, doctors made most of the decisions. After the 1970's and the passage of the Patient Bill of Rights, patients began to make their own decisions about treatment much more often

C.   Two famous Supreme Court cases dealt with whether it was right to stop a treatment that was keeping someone alive and also considered who could make decisions for a patient who was not able to make decisions for herself

   1.   Karen Ann Quinlan case-1976. A young woman was in a persistent vegetative state (PVS), which is a chronic condition like a coma in which a person does not have higher level brain function. This means the person cannot speak or move purposefully; does not respond to stimulation; must have all care done for him or her. Karen Ann's father wanted her removed from the ventilator, but the hospital refused because Karen Ann had never made her wishes about treatment known. The Court ruled that the hospital should remove Karen from the ventilator. She lived for many years after it was removed, breathing on her own, but being fed by a tube

   2.   Nancy Beth Cruzan case-1990. A young woman was in a PVS and her family wanted her feeding tube removed. The judge learned that Nancy had often told her friends that she would not want to live on machines or with tubes. Based on these statements, the judge ruled that the feeding tube should be removed. After the tube was removed, Ms. Cruzan died

D.   Another case more recently reminds us that these issues have not been resolved even though more than twenty years have passed since the first case

   1.   Terri Schiavo case-1998. A young woman who had been dieting collapsed and suffered a cardiac arrest. After several attempts at resuscitation she responded but her brain was likely without oxygen for a long time. As a result, she lost her ability to speak, think, and move and was diagnosed as being in a PVS. After many attempts at rehabilitation, she was admitted to a nursing home on a feeding tube. Her husband believed strongly that she would not want to live this way, but her parents disagreed. The case was in the Florida courts and received great attention from state and national lawmakers, clergy, and the public. Her feeding tube was finally removed and she died shortly after

E.   The field called bioethics started in the early 1970's when people began to study and explore the issues related to the use of medical technology and who should make decisions about when it should be used

F.   Based on these trends, healthcare ethics, laws, and practices changed

   1.   Adults now have the right to decide what will happen to their bodies (in other words, they now have autonomy)

2. States passed laws in which people could state, before they became too ill, what they would want as far as treatments in certain situations (e.g., whether they would want to be resuscitated and placed on a ventilator if they had terminal cancer)

3. In 1991, a federal law was passed called the Patient Self Determination Act (PSDA)

    a) PSDA says that all patients in hospitals, nursing homes, and hospice and home care programs who receive money from the United States government must be told that they have the right to make decisions about what medical treatment they want or do not want

    b) Patients now have the right to accept or refuse any treatment, even if the person would die if he or she refuses a particular treatment

    c) As part of the PSDA, hospitals, hospices, nursing homes, and home care programs must encourage their patients to make out some kind of advance directive (such as a living will, durable power of attorney for healthcare, or healthcare proxy)

VII. The Ethics of End-of-Life Decision-Making

A. The PSDA and other laws help set the standard that people have a right to have their wishes honored even if they can no longer speak for themselves

B. Many conditions can prevent people from telling us what their wishes are, such as

    1. Persistent vegetative state (PVS), coma

    2. Dementia

    3. Stroke

    4. Cancer

C. Advance directives allow people to document their wishes for treatment in these circumstances

D. There are two major types of advance directives

    1. Living will

        a) A person writes down the kinds of treatments he or she would want or not want in certain conditions, e.g., if the person were terminally ill or in a coma, or had a condition such as Alzheimer's disease

        b) On this form, a person can say that he or she wants (or does not want) treatments such as antibiotics, tube feedings, CPR or kidney dialysis

        c) People can also include issues related to pain medications and other drugs

> *Advance directives allow people to document their wishes for future healthcare decisions in the event they can no longer speak for themselves.*

    2. Durable power of attorney for healthcare (DPOA-HC) or healthcare proxy

        a) A person names someone whom she or he trusts to make healthcare decisions when or if the person becomes unable to make her or his own decisions

        b) The person named as DPOA-HC makes decisions only when the patient becomes unable to make his or her own decisions

        c) Until that time, the patient makes his or her own treatment decisions

E. Respecting autonomy: patient decision-making and giving informed consent
    1. Patient decision-making includes the right to accept or refuse any treatment, even if refusing the treatment will result in death
    2. When a decision must be made about a particular treatment, the healthcare team must give the patient (or the appointed decision-maker) complete information about the patient's condition, choices about treatment, and pros and cons of treatment
    3. When the patient, or the appointed decision-maker, has all the information, he or she then must decide which, if any of the treatments are desired
    4. Agreeing or not agreeing to a treatment after being given all the information about the person's condition and possible treatment is referred to as giving informed consent
    5. The healthcare team must determine if the patient is able to make decisions; just because the patient has dementia or another condition that limits his or her ability to think and express wishes, the team should not assume that the person cannot make decisions[3,5]
    6. If the person is not able to make decisions, it needs to be decided who can make decisions for that person
        a) If the person can understand and respond, we must first talk to the patient
        b) If the person cannot understand, we try to find out if the person ever did an advance directive
            i.   If the patient completed a living will, the healthcare team should do whatever the will says the person wants
            ii. If the patient named someone to be the durable power of attorney or healthcare proxy, the team needs to help that person to make good treatment decisions based on the patient's medical condition, how long the patient is expected to live, and what is best for the patient based on what has been done for patients in similar situations
F. Common end-of-life treatment decisions
    1. Specific treatment choices at the end of life include the following
        a) CPR
        b) Breathing machine, called a ventilator
        c) Whether to transfer the patient to the hospital
        d) Feeding tubes
        e) Intravenous therapy and intravenous hydration
        f) Antibiotics
        g) Diagnostic tests
        h) Blood transfusions
    2. Each decision requires that the patient or other decision-maker understand
        a) What the patient's goals are
        b) What kinds of things are important to the patient, or the patient's values
        c) The patient's diagnosis and prognosis, or what exactly the patient's disease is, how it will worsen, and an educated guess about how long the patient can live

3. Decision-making is an ongoing process and even after a decision is made, the team should continue talking with the patient and family about the patient's condition and their choices for care

VIII. Other Ethical Issues at the End of Life[3,4]

A. Confidentiality: keeping patients' personal information private
B. Withholding or withdrawing treatment
   1. Legally, ethically and medically, there is no difference between not starting a treatment (withholding) and stopping it once it has been started (withdrawing)
   2. Many people feel that there is an emotional difference between stopping a treatment and not starting a treatment at all; for many people, it is harder emotionally to withdraw (stop) therapy once it has been started
   3. Starting a treatment, such as an IV or a feeding tube, to see if it helps a person, and then stopping it if the person does not get any better is often a good idea (this is called a time-limited trial); trials may give families peace of mind because they know they tried everything possible, even if it did not work
C. Administering pain medications[6]
   1. Healthcare workers are legally required to treat their patients' pain
   2. If a person is in severe pain, it is unethical not to use strong medications, such as morphine, to relieve the pain
   3. Some nurses and physicians fear that giving morphine and similar drugs can cause the patient to die
   4. There is no proof that giving morphine can speed up the dying process; however, the nurse should give the pain medication even if it might make a person die sooner because there is a duty to relieve suffering and pain
D. Providing artificial food and water[3]
   1. Loss of appetite is a common symptom at the end of life and often is distressing to families
   2. Food is often seen as a symbol of love and nurturing; we can help families explore other ways to comfort the patient e.g., by giving mouth care or gently rubbing the patient's hand with lotion
   3. We can encourage patients to take food and water, but we cannot force them
   4. Artificial food (liquid given through a feeding tube) and water (given through a feeding tube or intravenous line) generally cause more discomfort when someone is near the end of life
   5. The team should give patients and families correct information to help them decide when they are asked to make decisions about using artificial feeding and fluids
   6. We should honor patients' and families' decisions about these therapies
E. Truth-telling[3,4]
   1. United States laws and medical ethics strongly encourage telling patients the truth about their conditions
   2. Healthcare workers sometimes think that patients will be upset if they hear bad news
   3. When doctors give patients bad news about their conditions, it must be done in a kind and sensitive manner

4. Patients who get bad news from their healthcare providers need emotional support and also need to feel they will be cared for, no matter what happens

5. Truth should be offered to patients, but not forced upon them

F. Assisted death[3,7]

1. Assisted death is a term that includes

   a) Euthanasia: acting to end the life of a patient to relieve the patient's suffering; also called "mercy killing;" it usually involves a doctor or a nurse giving a deadly injection to the patient

   b) Assisted suicide: providing a person with a medication knowing that the person plans to kill himself or herself by taking an overdose of the medication

2. Euthanasia: legal in the Netherlands, but it is not legal anywhere in the United States

3. As of 1997, assisted suicide has been practiced legally in Oregon; in 2008, a similar law was passed in Washington State; assisted suicide usually involves a doctor writing a prescription for a lethal medication (that a patient must be able to take); assisted suicide currently (as of January 2009) is illegal in every other state besides Oregon and Washington

4. Assisted death is a controversial and emotional issue

5. Giving patients strong medications to ease their pain is not euthanasia or assisted suicide

IX. Cultural Issues in Ethics[2]

A. People from different cultures and religions often have differing opinions about the morality of certain healthcare issues and treatments

B. At the end of life, these differing views often focus on

1. Use of feeding tubes

2. Whether to tell patients the truth about their conditions

3. Assisted suicide or euthanasia

4. Whether or not to fill out an advance directive

5. The use of life-saving actions such as CPR or ventilation

6. Who should make decisions; in some cultures, the family, a male spouse, or the eldest male child, makes decisions even if the patient is able to do so

C. Healthcare workers must learn about and respect the views of people from different cultures and religions if they are going to care for them appropriately[2,3]

X. Summary

A. Ethics gives us guidance about whether a particular action is right or wrong

B. Many important ethical issues develop at the end of life, especially about how people make decisions about treatment

C. Problems occur when people disagree about what is moral; these disagreements cause ethical dilemmas

D. Ethical dilemmas often are very challenging

E. Ethical dilemmas should be dealt with by the entire team, not just one person

F. Nursing Assistants are part of the healthcare team and their role in dealing with ethical issues is as a team member

G. Sometimes, ethics committees help healthcare workers resolve ethical dilemmas

H. If you feel distress over an ethical problem at work, you should talk with your supervisor, chaplain, or other trusted person

CITED REFERENCES

1. Carter J, Chichin ER. *Palliative care in the nursing home.* In: Morrison RS, Meier DE, eds. Geriatric palliative care. New York, NY: Oxford University Press; 2003:357-375.

2. Farber Post L, Blustein J, Dubler NN. *Handbook for Healthcare Ethics Committees.* Baltimore, MD: Johns Hopkins University Press; 2007.

3. American Association of Colleges of Nursing (AACN) and the City of Hope National Medical Center. Module 4: Goals of care and ethical Issues at the end of life. *End-of-Life Nursing Education Consortium (ELNEC) - Geriatric*; 2008.

4. Beauchamp T, Childress J, *Principles of Biomedical Ethics*, 6th ed. New York, NY: Oxford University Press; 2008.

5. American Geriatrics Society. *Making Treatment Decisions for Incapacitated Elderly with Advance Directives.* Accessed October 1, 2008. Available from URL: www.americangeriatrics.org/products/positionpapers/treatdec.shtml.

6. *The Ethics of Opiate use Within Palliative Care.* (Position Statement). Pittsburgh, PA: Hospice and Palliative Nurses Association, 2008. Accessed January 9, 2009. Available at: http://www.hpna.org/DisplayPage.aspx?Title=Position%20Statements

7. *Legalization of Assisted Suicide.* (Position Statement). Pittsburgh, PA: Hospice and Palliative Nurses Association, 2006. Accessed January 9, 2009. Available at: http://www.hpna.org/DisplayPage.aspx?Title=Position%20Statements

CHAPTER 5
COMMUNICATING AT THE END OF LIFE

Joanne E. Sheldon, MEd, MSN, RN, CHPN®

Original Author
Mary Ersek, RN, PhD, FAAN, Marty Richards, MSW, LICSW

I. Basic Concepts of Communication[1,2]

A. Definition of communication

1. Exchanging information that shares meaning

2. Involves two parts

a) Sending information by speaking/signals

b) Receiving information through listening and/or observing

3. Can be verbal and/or nonverbal

B. Verbal communication

1. Words that a person says

2. Sounds that a person makes such as moans, groans, sighs

3. May be garbled or difficult to understand

4. When a person loses their ability to speak due to aphasia or other problems, they usually continue to understand what is spoken to them and will respond in their usual manner

5. Never assume that one cannot communicate using words nor that they might not understand what another is saying

C. Nonverbal communication

1. Ways of communicating with another without using words, e.g.,

a) Posture, how a person sits or stands

b) Gestures

c) How a person moves

d) Facial expressions

e) Tone of voice

f) Appearance such as clothing, hair, jewelry, etc.

g) Use or non use of eye contact

h) Touching or lack of comfort with being touched

i. Can communicate support, respect, and care although touch also can offend or threaten some people, and invade their personal space

> ❖ *93% of communication is non-verbal*
>
> ❖ *7% of communication is verbal*

    ii. Allow the other person to take the lead in showing you whether or not it is okay to touch; observe a person's response to initial touch to decide if this communication style is acceptable

  2. Silence and communication

    a) Provides a chance for another person to be heard and to think about what he/she might want to share

    b) Is a way of "being present"

    c) May be comforting

    d) Does not necessarily mean that the other does not want to talk; might mean that they are thinking deeply, experiencing pain or feeling very emotional

    e) May also indicate that the person is unsure what to say at a certain moment; it is important to give someone time to respond

    f) Learn to be comfortable with silence; this comfort is a skill to practice

D. Creating an environment that encourages effective communication

  1. Position yourself so that the person can see you

    a) Allow the person to see you before you speak or touch him/her

    b) Be at eye level; standing above a person to talk may show an attitude of power

    c) Sit so that the light is not directly in the face of either of you so that you can easily see the face of the other; the other person may need to read your lips

    d) Locate or create a quiet and a private place to speak

  2. Turn off the television or radio

  3. Ask the person if you should close the door for privacy

  4. Turn off or mute your cell phone and pager

  5. If the person has hearing difficulties sit close; insert hearing aid, if necessary

  6. Arrange adequate time to be with this person – do not rush

  7. Call the person by the name he/she prefers

  8. Avoid distracting behaviors such as pacing, frowning, chewing gum

  9. Wear your name badge where it can be seen so that the person knows who you are

E. Listening – a basic communication skill

  1. Listening is the process of receiving, paying attention to, and making meaning about what another person is communicating

  2. Focus on the other person

  3. Stop talking

  4. Allow time for the other person to speak

  5. Be aware of any cultural issues, e.g., is it okay to make eye contact or to touch the person

  6. Use nonverbal communication effectively

    a) Lean toward the person

    b) Nod your head

    c) Do not cross your arms

     d) Acknowledge what the person is telling you by making comments as, "I see" or "tell me more"

     e) If you do not understand what the person is saying, ask for an explanation, but do not interrupt

     f) Be patient; allow time in between sentences

F. The skill of speaking

  1. Speak slowly and clearly, but do not talk down to the person

  2. Use clear words and simple sentences

  3. Do not use slang words, provide an explanation when using abbreviations and medical terminology, e.g., instead of saying you are a *CNA*, say you are a *Certified Nursing Assistant* or instead of saying you are going to *take* their *BP*, say you are going to *check* their *blood pressure*

  4. Repeat ideas several times, if necessary

  5. Be aware of your nonverbal language: does it match your verbal communication? For example, are you saying, "Take your time" yet you are talking fast and moving quickly, implying the person should hurry

  6. Do not talk too loudly or softly; ask if the person can hear you; if not, talk a bit louder and ask him again; avoid shouting

  7. Do not raise your voice just because the person is older or speaks another language

G. Written materials for communication

  1. Use large simple print with dark letters on white paper

  2. Use simple drawings and pictures

  3. Use simple words and short sentences

  4. Give the person time to read the material and then discuss it to assure understanding

  5. Review material with the person on a regular basis

II. **Cultural Differences in Communication** (also see Chapter 6) [1,2]

A. Styles of communication vary with different cultures e.g.,

  1. Use eye contact

  2. Use of touch

B. Who receives information; The patient? The spouse? The eldest son? Someone else?

C. Ask the patient and/or family if they have preferences on how to communicate

  1. Observe how family members interact with one another

     a) Do they speak directly and to the point?

     b) Do they talk in very general terms?

     c) Do they openly ask questions and answer them?

     d) Do they hesitate to ask questions in front of the patient?

     e) Do they talk openly and honestly about illness and death?

     f) Do they speak with their eyes or face?

     g) Do they use their hands and arms?

     h) Do they sit or stand very quietly?

D. Be aware that words may mean different things to people
   1. Your understanding of the meaning of one word may mean something different to another person (family, faith, care)
   2. Avoid abbreviations; e.g., "PRN", "DNR" or jargon, e.g., "terminal restlessness" as they are often misunderstood
   3. Do not assume that you know what a person means; ask them what they mean if you are unsure
E. Allow time for the other person to ask you questions
F. Learn if the person's culture approves of telling a dying person that, "It is okay to let go"
G. Follow the patient's needs and wishes for his care, not the family's
H. If an interpreter is needed, use a person trained as a medical interpreter rather than family members

III. Gender Differences in Communication[1,2]
A. Men and women tend to communicate differently when sharing information and feelings
B. Men and women of various cultures may do things differently; e.g., in some Arabic cultures, men do not usually provide childcare

IV. Age[1,2]
A. Consider the person's developmental stage
B. Make sure they are able to understand the terminology used such as "terminal" or "actively dying"
C. Elders expect to receive respect in words and action
D. Ask each person how she or he prefers to be addressed, e.g., Mr. Jones, Bob, or Reverend Smith
E. Be aware of sensory losses, such as hearing loss, that occur in old age and may make communication more difficult

V. Identifying Your Own Communication Style[1,2]
A. All of us have different ways of expressing ourselves; differences in communication styles are not bad or good, they just are
B. Think about your own style and how it affects your actions and people's responses to you
C. Do not label people because their communication style differs from yours; e.g., someone who is quiet may be labeled as withdrawn; someone who is assertive and has a loud voice can be seen as pushy or threatening
D. The healthcare team should build on the strengths of each member's communication style
E. Learn to give honest but helpful feedback to other team members about their communication style

VI. Effective Communication: Special Issues in Working with the Dying[1,2]
A. Difficulties in communicating with dying patients

1. Cultural and societal issues
   a) People often are uneasy talking about death
   b) Many people have not spent time with people who are dying
2. Patients' and families' feelings (see next section on Dealing with Conflict)
3. Concerns of the care provider
   a) Not knowing what to say or not knowing "the answer"
   b) Fear of making a mistake and upsetting the patient or family
   c) Fear of showing emotions
   d) Feeling uncomfortable about being around people who are upset, sad, or angry
   e) Personal fear of dying
4. Conditions that make communication difficult, such as stroke, dementia, hearing and vision problems, sleepiness, and confusion

B. Common patients' and families' feelings that affect communication
   1. Fear of
      a) Pain and other symptoms
      b) Dying alone
      c) Receiving poor care, or not receiving the care they need
      d) Losing the ability to think and express oneself
      e) Losing control
      f) Dying process, death, afterlife
      g) Losing relationships
      h) Losing one's identity as a mother, daughter, employee, etc.
      i) Money problems, loss of income
      j) Being a burden
   2. Anger at
      a) Effects of the illness
      b) People who do not seem to understand
      c) Loss of job and income
      d) Loss of plans and dreams
      e) The fact that their loved one is leaving them
   3. Guilt (especially families)
      a) For what they should have done
      b) About what they did in the past
      c) About needing time away from their loved one or for not being there more
      d) For losing their temper
      e) About unresolved relationships
      f) About not being able to care for the dying person on their own
   4. Sadness
      a) Can be overwhelming
      b) Occurs often and can get worse with each new loss

5. Confusion
    a) Inability to keep up with changes
    b) Inability to think clearly
    c) Difficulty making decisions
6. Hopelessness and helplessness
    a) Feeling that a loss of control
    b) Sensing there is nothing that can be done
    c) Feeling abandoned
    d) Feeling alone
7. Love and joy
    a) Laughter and joy can occur in the midst of suffering and loss
    b) Humor can be an effective way to cope

C. Necessary communication skills
    1. Sometimes, we worry so much about saying the RIGHT thing that we say nothing at all...that is okay, being "present" is important
    2. "Join the patient on the journey"
    3. Take the lead from patients and families about what they want to share with you
    4. You do not have to have all the answers; it is okay to say that you do not know the answer
    5. Encourage reminiscing[1]
        a) Reminiscing is remembering and talking about what happened in the past; includes telling stories about a person's life
        b) Helps patients and families to see that a person's life has meaning and is important
        c) Helps to take the focus off their problems
        d) Be ready and willing to listen to the sadness that may come with reminiscing
    6. Important messages to communicate[1]
        a) "I will listen to you"
        b) "I will be honest and truthful with you"
        c) "I will not abandon you"
        d) "I value you as a person"
        e) "I will respect your values and goals and help you to achieve those goals as much as I am able"
        f) "I will give you every chance to ask questions. If I do not know the answer to your question, I will try to find someone who does"
        g) "I accept that you will at times be sad, frightened, or angry. I will not turn away or avoid you when you are experiencing these emotions"
        h) "When caring for you or your loved one, I will ask myself, 'What would I want if this were my family member?'"

> *Sometimes, we worry so much about saying the RIGHT thing that we say nothing at all...that is okay, being "present" is important*

    7.   Make sure there is a good match between verbal and nonverbal messages; e.g., telling the patient that they can trust you, but failing to answer their call light is confusing communication

D. Timing
    1.   Make sure that someone is physically comfortable as you begin to talk with him or her
    2.   Be aware of the times that patients want to talk about certain things; respect their wishes when they do not want to talk; use their timetable, not your own

E. Asking questions
    1.   Remember that patients and families have limited energy for questions
    2.   Limit questions by focusing on the patient's or family's concerns; do not ask questions if you really do not need or want to know the answer
    3.   Questions should show that you are really interested in the patient's situation; respect the privacy of people's feelings
    4.   If you need to ask a sensitive question, explain why you are asking the question
    5.   Use open-ended questions; e.g., ask, "How did that make you feel?" instead of, "Did that make you feel sad?"

F. Providing hope without making false assurances[6]
    1.   How you communicate with patients and families can increase or decrease hope
    2.   Ways to support patients' and families' hope
        a) Ask people about their goals and help them to achieve them
        b) Be present, even at sad or difficult times
        c) Show a person respect no matter how they look or act
        d) Provide excellent care to relieve suffering
        e) Help patients and families express their spirituality

G. Patients' communication at the end of life[3]
    1.   Often, dying patients and their families want to share memories and emotions
    2.   Sometimes people use symbols to express their feelings or their understandings about their own living and dying; this is known as "nearing death awareness"; e.g., patients may
        a) Talk about meeting and talking with others who have died before them
        b) Insist that a dead relative or friend is "waiting for me"
        c) Talk about needing to get "a ticket for the train"
        d) Messages may indicate that the person knows that death is near and that he or she is ready to die
    3.   Some patients may need to talk with others to settle relationships and say they are sorry for past actions

H. Educating and supporting families and patients in terminal illness
    1.   Help people understand the importance of sharing with each other at end of life
    2.   Educate and support patients and families by role modeling effective communication skills
    3.   Use written materials so the patient and family have a resource to review
    4.   Explain nearing-death awareness and help families recognize and honor it

VII. Dealing with Conflict[2,4]

A. The crisis of a terminal illness can bring issues to the surface and result in family conflicts; if you get caught right in the middle of it, remember
   1. There are many sides to every situation
   2. Do not take sides
   3. You see only a snapshot in the whole moving picture of the family's interactions
   4. Anger may be directed at other family members because they are "safe" and patients know that they will be forgiven as part of unconditional love that exists in some families
   5. Grief can be expressed as anger
   6. Anger may be directed at healthcare team members

B. Dealing with patient or family anger directed at healthcare provider
   1. Tips for managing your own responses
      a) Take an emotional step back from the situation; if you can, physically get away from the situation
      b) Think about your emotions. What exactly are you feeling? Anger? Fear? Sadness? Something else?
      c) Do any of the emotions you are feeling show themselves in your actions? How?
      d) Talk with other team members about how you are feeling; together, try to figure out what the conflict is about and who is involved
      e) Talk with the other people involved in the conflict; make a plan for dealing with the conflict or disagreement
      f) Always use "I" statements, e.g., "I am trying to understand what you would like me to do," or "I feel uncomfortable when you raise your voice"
   2. When you communicate with someone who is angry or distressed, remember the following
      a) Recognize frustrating and frightening situations; put yourself in the person's situation. How would you feel? How would you want to be treated?
      b) Treat the person with respect by using active listening skills; let the person express their anger
      c) Answer the person's questions clearly; if you cannot answer the questions, ask the nurse or other team member to answer them
      d) Keep the person informed; tell the person what you are going to do and why
      e) Do not keep the person waiting for long periods; address the person's questions and concerns as quickly as possible
      f) Stay calm; recognize that the person may be frustrated or frightened by the situation
      g) Recognize that families and patients need to express their grief and frustration; remember that anger is a normal part of the grieving process
      h) Do not argue with or touch the person
      i) Protect yourself from violent behaviors, e.g., stand far enough away from the person so that they cannot kick or hit you, stand close to a door or other exit
      j) Report the person's behavior to the nurse or other team member

VIII. Summary

A. Communication is an exchange of ideas between the sender and the receiver

B. 93% of communication is non-verbal and 7% of communication of verbal

C. Often, dying patients and their families want to share memories and emotions

D. Learn to be comfortable with silence as it is a skill and it is a way of being present

E. It is important to role model effective communication skills

CITED REFERENCES

1. American Association of Colleges of Nursing (AACN) and the City of Hope National Medical Center. Module 6: Communication. *End-of-Life Nursing Education Consortium (ELNEC) - Geriatric,* 2008.

2. Edwards M, Ersek M, ed. *Nursing Assistant End-of-life Care Computerized Education Program (NA-CEP).* Pittsburgh, PA: Hospice and Palliative Nurses Association; 2006.

3. Callanan M, Kelley P. *Final Gifts: Understanding the Special Awareness, Needs & Communications of the Dying.* New York, NY: Bantam Books; 1992.

4. Sorrentino SA, Kelly RT. *Mosby's Textbook for Nursing Assistants. 7th Ed.* St. Louis, MO:Mosby; 2007;52-71.

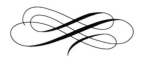

CHAPTER 6
CULTURAL CONSIDERATIONS AT THE END OF LIFE

Jeanne Martinez, RN, MPH, CHPN®, Mary Ersek, RN, PhD, FAAN

Original Author
Sarah A. Wilson, RN, PhD

I. **Culture**

   A. Definitions

      1. The values, beliefs, and practices of a particular group that are learned and shared and that guide a person's thinking, decisions, and actions in a patterned way[1]

      2. Culture is all the beliefs, practices, customs, rituals, and values we learn, first from our families, then in school, the community, and other social organizations such as church[2]

   B. Characteristics of culture[2,3,4]

      1. Universally: all humans have a culture or cultures that influence them

      2. Shared by members of a cultural group; it is what makes them a group

      3. Changes slowly over time

      4. Defines roles and responsibilities

      5. Most often associated with a particular ethnic group (e.g., Hispanic culture), but may also refer to religious group, age group, or sexual orientation; e.g., we may talk about Jewish culture, culture of the elderly, or gay community

      6. People may belong to more than one cultural group, e.g., a 70-year-old black woman, who is a Jehovah Witness would belong to the elderly, black, and religious group cultures

      7. One culture is not better than another culture; they are just different

> *One culture is not better than another culture; they are just different!*

   C. Concepts related to culture[2,3]

      1. Ethnicity or ethnic group

         a) Refers to a sense of shared personhood; things people have in common

         b) The common feature that defines the ethnic group may be geographic region, language, traditions, values, or interest in homeland

      2. Acculturation

         a) Process of adapting to another culture

         b) People immigrating to the United States may give up certain habits or practices that were common in their home culture and adopt habits that are common in the United States

      3. Race[4]

         a) Refers to a group of people having similar ancestors and physical features who sometimes share a culture (e.g, American Indian, African-American,

Caucasian, and Asian)

b) Different than culture

c) Has been used to put people into groups and to treat certain groups unfairly

d) Racism: belief that race is the key factor in determining human qualities and abilities, and that one race is superior to another

4. Diversity[4]

a) Refers to the differences among people

b) Includes race, gender, language, physical characteristics, disability, sexual orientation, economic status, parental status, education, geographic origin, profession, lifestyle, and religion

5. Stereotype

a) Mental picture that is held in common by a group and that represents an oversimplified opinion or prejudiced attitude of another group

b) Expecting people to act in a certain way without seeing that people are individuals

c) Some examples include the assumptions that blondes are dumb, American Indians drink too much, and older adults have poor memories

d) Are usually negative ideas or judgments about members of a certain ethnic, racial or other group

6. Prejudice

a) Negative beliefs about a group of people

b) Making judgments about people, usually negative

D. Changing population in the United States[5]

1. United States is a collection of many different cultural groups and is called a multicultural society

2. If immigration trends continue, the U.S. population will have a greater variety of cultural groups; over 50% of the population will be a culture other than white, non-Hispanic

3. According to 2004 census projections[4], by 2010, the U.S. population will be:

a) 15.5% Hispanic or Latino

b) 13% Black or African American

c) 5% Asian and Pacific Islander

d) 3% Native American, Alaskan Native, Pacific Islander, or 2 or more races

E. Why study culture?

1. To understand how people view the world and what they value

2. To learn more about our own culture

3. To understand how culture influences a person's beliefs about

a) Health and illness

b) What causes illness

c) What should be done about illness

d) Where to get advice about illness

4. To improve our ability to interact and communicate with others; to be nonjudgmental and good listeners

5. To provide care that is sensitive to a person's cultural beliefs and values
6. To help us realize that not everyone in a cultural group is the same; factors that may influence these differences are
   a) Age
   b) Length of time the person has been in the country
   c) Education
   d) Income or socioeconomic level
   e) Religion
   f) Geographic location in current country
7. To help us see how similar we are, despite some differences

II. Cultural Competence

A. Definitions
   1. *Cultural sensitivity* is an awareness of differences among cultural groups
   2. *Cultural competence* is a combination of knowledge, attitudes, and skills that helps people better talk and interact with people who are different from them

> *Cultural sensitivity is an awareness of differences among cultural groups.*

B. To give culturally competent care you must[4]
   1. Develop an awareness of your own culture and how it influences your attitudes, communication styles and beliefs
   2. Demonstrate knowledge and understanding of the patient's culture, health-related needs, and meanings of health and illness
   3. Accept and respect cultural differences
   4. Not assume that your patient's beliefs and values are the same as your own
   5. Resist attitudes such as "different is not as good"
   6. Be open to and comfortable with cultural encounters
   7. Adapt care to match the patient's cultural beliefs, values, and practices

C. Culturally competent healthcare workers[2]
   1. Are willing to learn
   2. Ask questions
   3. Keep open mind; avoid making assumptions and judging others
   4. Learn from mistakes
   5. Appreciate differences in people
   6. Recognize that building relationships takes time and energy

> *Cultural competence is a combination of knowledge, attitude, and skills that help you communicate with people of diverse groups*

D. To develop cultural skills, use the LEARN model[6]
   1. L - listen to the patient
   2. E - explain what you hear the patient saying
   3. A - acknowledge differences between the patient and the healthcare provider
   4. R - recognize that differences exist
   5. N - negotiate with the patient to develop a plan, make recommendations that incorporate the patient's view

III. Cultural Identity

A. All cultures have similar components, or parts; these parts make up a person's cultural identity. Fong's CONFHER model is used to identify key aspects of cultural identity[7]

B. CONFHER includes

1. C - Communication
   a) Does the patient speak English? Does the patient understand common health terms such as "pain" or "fever"?
   b) Is an interpreter needed?
   c) What nonverbal behaviors are acceptable to the patients and family? e.g., Native Americans tend to avoid eye contact and value silence; Mexican Americans often value closeness and touch; Japanese Americans may bow head to show respect when greeting someone

2. O - Orientation
   a) How does the patient identify himself? Do they identify with a particular group (e.g., Asian, African) or ethnic group (e.g., Chinese, Korean, etc.)?
   b) Where were they born? How long did they live there?
   c) Ask about the person's ideas about: the relationship between humans and nature, time orientation: (present, past, or future oriented)

3. N - Nutrition
   a) Includes food, food preferences, and taboos
   b) Food has meaning for most people and may be associated with certain events or celebrations, e.g., people may have special food for Christmas, Chanukah, or birthdays
   c) Food is a source of comfort and love. Avoid making assumptions that people eat certain foods based on their ethnicity
   d) Ask people if there are any foods that they must avoid, e.g., eating pork is not acceptable for a Jewish or Muslim person

4. F - Family relationships
   a) Who is in the family? What is the patient's definition of family?
   b) Who is the head of the household?
   c) What is the role of women, the elderly, and children?
   d) Family dynamics refers to family relationships and how the family gets things done; questions to ask include - How are decisions made? Is it important to have family present when someone is sick? For example in many traditional Korean families, the eldest adult son is expected to make the health-care decisions for an aged parent

5. H - Health and health beliefs
   a) Refer to an attitude that influences health behavior; it is what the person believes about health and the causes of health problems or disease
   b) Questions related to health beliefs include
      i. What does the patient do to stay healthy?
      ii. Who does the patient consult for a health problem: family, physician or nurse, or other healer?
      iii. How does the patient explain illness?

      iv.   Is illness explained by a disease model, e.g., a virus, or is disease caused by an imbalance in the body, or evil spirits?

      v.   How does the patient react to health problems? Is the person stoic and tries to not to show any discomfort or emotion? Or does the person openly display emotions and discomfort?

      vi.   Example of health and health beliefs: Mexican Americans may believe that disease is caused by an imbalance between the person and environment; they may consult with a Curandismo, or traditional healer, who attempts healing by use of special prayers and rituals

6.   E - Education

    a)   Education refers to

      i.   The ways in which a person finds it easiest to learn something, e.g., by reading a manual or watching a video

      ii.   Completion of a program of learning; e.g., high school, college

    b)   Questions to ask about education include

      i.   How does the patient learn best: Printed material? Visual aids? Auditory aids? By watching and doing?

      ii.   How much formal education did the patient complete?

7.   R - Religion

    a)   May include spiritual beliefs of participation in religious practices

    b)   Questions to consider

      i.   What is the patient's religious preference?

      ii.   Does the patient have any religious beliefs or restrictions that have an impact on health and healthcare? e.g., Jehovah's Witness do not believe in blood transfusions

      iii.   If the patient and/or family do not identify with a particular religion, what helps them to find meaning in life? What rituals are important?

IV. Culture at the End of Life (EOL)[8]

A.   Although death is universal to all people and all cultures, culture affects many aspects of dying, e.g.,

   1.   How EOL decisions are made

   2.   How symptoms are expressed and managed

   3.   Death and mourning rituals

B.   Culture and EOL decision-making

   1.   EOL care often reflects American values, which includes the following ideas

    a)   People have the right to make decisions about their healthcare

    b)   People should be told the truth about their illness or condition so they can make informed decisions

    c)   People should have control over their life and death

    d)   People should express their wishes about the kind of care they want at the EOL by completing forms such as living wills (see Chapter 4)

   2.   Many cultural groups in the United States do not share these values; instead they may believe that

    a)   Telling patients the truth about their illness takes away the patient's hope; the patient should be protected from bad news; talking about bad things, such as death, may actually make those bad things happen sooner

b) The family's role is to make decisions for the patient; the patient, especially the older patient, should not have to make healthcare decisions

c) Illness and death are part of the natural rhythms of the universe; humans should not try to change the natural course of things

3. Examples of multicultural views of EOL decision making

a) Asian and Pacific Island cultures often believe the family should make the healthcare decisions for the older, dying patient; a person should not be told he or she has a terminal illness; protecting someone from the truth allows him or her to maintain hope

b) Native Americans may believe truth telling violates their traditions and talking about bad things makes them happen

4. Advance directives, such as living wills, and "No Code" orders, may be viewed by some cultural groups as denying treatment to the ill person; this is especially true for African-Americans and people with disabilities, who have been mistreated in our healthcare system

> *Healthcare workers should ask the patient and family if they have any practices, traditions, or rituals that are important to them when a loved one dies.*

C. Culture and EOL symptom management

1. Pain

a) Culture influences how people respond to pain and the emotions they express; e.g., some cultures encourage open expression of pain and emotion, whereas other cultures do not approve of expressing emotion and pain openly

b) May be seen as life affirming, the body is fighting back

c) May be viewed as a punishment

d) Response to pain may vary by gender; for some cultures, it is a sign of weakness for a male to express pain

2. Nutrition

a) Food is associated with living and is a source of comfort; food and fluids are essential to life

b) Decisions about artificial nutrition and hydration are controversial; for some families and individuals, not providing artificial food and fluids is cruel and results in starving the person to death

c) Cultural groups may have beliefs specific to food and hydration: e.g., Chinese often define a "good death" as being surrounded by family and having a full stomach

D. Cultural variations in death rituals

1. Death rituals include preparations for death, mourning, and burial practices

2. Examples of typical cultural and religious variations in death rituals (also see Chapters 7 and 8)

a) Orthodox Jews: bury the deceased as soon as possible, even on the same day of the death, but no more than two nights after the death. After-death rituals occur after the burial. Shiva, is a seven-day mourning period when mourners do not work, mirrors are covered, and no activity is permitted that would divert attention from the deceased; after Shiva, mourning period begins and varies based on who has died; e.g., mourning for a relative is 30 days and one year for a parent; tombstone is erected one year after death

    b) Mexican Americans hold elaborate ceremonies; e.g., a Velorio, to honor the dead; ceremonies lasts for days

    c) Muslims face Mecca when approaching death and recite passages from the Holy Qur'an

    d) Traditionally, Hmong believe a person should be dressed in the finest traditional Hmong clothing so he or she will enter the next world well dressed

    e) Native Americans view death as a natural process; a death song is sung that is a summary of a person's life and accomplishments

    f) Chinese believe the most important obligation in life is to bury the dead and honor ancestors with religious rites

    g) The time for mourning is short in the American culture: there is no clearly defined period of mourning; people are expected to "get on with living": within a week or so of death, all but the closest relatives have returned to their usual lives; people often are alone to grieve

3. Healthcare workers should ask families if they have any practices that are important to them when a loved one dies. *Do not make assumptions about what the person or family wants*

4. Healthcare workers *must not force their own religious or cultural beliefs on patients and families*

V. Summary

A. The United States is a diverse country with people from many different cultural groups

B. Culture has a significant influence on dying and death. What people think and believe about dying and death is influenced by culture

C. Healthcare workers need knowledge of culture to provide culturally appropriate EOL care

D. The process of becoming culturally competent begins with examining your biases, and by being willing to learn and ask questions

E. Healthcare workers must not assume that all members of a group share the same beliefs and values about EOL care. Ask the patient and family about their values and practices

F. Do not force your beliefs on others

> *Healthcare workers must not force their own religious or cultural beliefs on patients and families.*

CITED REFERENCES

1. Leininger M. *Transcultural Nursing: Concepts, Theories and Practices.* New York, NY: John Wiley & Sons; 1978.

2. Purnell LD, Paulanka BJ, eds. *Transcultural Healthcare: A Culturally Competent Approach.* 3rd ed. Philadelphia, PA: F.A. Davis; 2008.

3. Spector RE. *Cultural Diversity in Health and Illness.* 7th ed. Upper Saddle River, NJ: Prentice Hall; 2008.

4. Purnell LD. Purnell Model of Cultural Competence. *Journal of Multicultural Nursing & Health.* 2005;11(2):7-15.

5. U.S. Census Bureau. *U.S. Interim Projections by Age, Sex, Race, and Hispanic Origin, 2004.* Available at: www.census.gov/ipc/www/usinterimproj/. Accessed November 3, 2008.

6. Berlin E, Fowkes WA. A teaching framework for cross-cultural healthcare. *Western Journal of Medicine.* 1982;139:934-938.

7. Fong CM. Ethnicity and nursing practice. *Topics in Clinical Nursing.* 1985;7(3):1-10.

8. American Association of Colleges of Nursing (AACN) and the City of Hope National Medical Center. Module 5: Cultural considerations in end-of-life care. *End-of-Life Nursing Education Consortium (ELNEC) Geriatric,* 2008.

ADDITIONAL RESOURCES AND REFERENCES

DiversityRx (website). Available at: www.diversityrx.org/. Accessed November 3, 2008.

Ethnomed (website). Available at: http://ethnomed.org/. Accessed November 3, 2008.

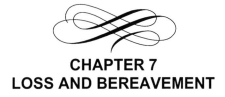

CHAPTER 7
LOSS AND BEREAVEMENT

Barbara Head, PhD, RN, CHPN®, ACSW

I. Introduction

A. Nursing Assistants develop close relationships with patients and their loved ones and can support and help patients and family members who are grieving both before and after the death

B. It is important to understand the grief process and know how to respond to grieving persons

C. To help grieving people, it is also important to understand your own feelings and beliefs and to practice good self care

II. Definitions

A. Grief

1. A person's response to a loss

2. Feelings and thoughts that are triggered when a person has a loss[1]

3. Often these feelings include emotional pain and sadness

4. Types of grief

   a) Anticipatory grief: grief that occurs before the actual death

   i. Often occurs among family members and friends who know their loved one is expected to die[2]

   ii. Does not necessarily lessen the experience of grief at the time of death

   b) Disenfranchised grief: a person's grief over a loss that is not recognized or accepted by others

   i. People who might experience disenfranchised grief include partners of HIV/AIDS patients, ex-spouses, mistresses or lovers and children who lose a stepparent[3]

   ii. The grieving person does not feel as though it is okay to openly express and talk about their feelings [4]

   c) Complicated grief:[3,5] a very intense grief reaction that lasts longer than a year may indicate the bereaved person may be having complicated grief; there are five types of complicated grief

   i. Chronic grief: grief that continues over a long period of time. The person is unable to recover from the loss and return to normal activities

   ii. Delayed grief: grief that is not expressed at the time of the loss. This may be because of other events or losses in the person's life that require time and energy

> Grief is a person's response to a loss.
>
> Mourning is the outward expression of a loss.

   iii. Exaggerated grief: symptoms of the grief are severe and may include nightmares, angry outbursts, extreme guilt, fear, and self-destructive behaviors such as attempted suicide, drug and alcohol abuse

   iv. Masked grief: bereaved person may show behaviors or symptoms such as depression or anger but they do not connect these problems to their loss

   v. Sudden grief: the death occurs suddenly and the grieving person has a difficult time accepting the reality of the loss. Often this occurs when the death is traumatic such as in the case of a murder, accident, military death, or suicide

 B. Loss

  1. Is experienced by both the dying patient and their family and loved ones throughout the time of the illness and death

  2. Patient losses include physical losses (loss of hair or change in body, loss of ability or strength), loss of their usual roles and activities, loss of relationships, and the loss of life as they now know it

  3. Family/friend losses include loss of the person as they once knew him or her, loss of their own usual activities as they care for the dying person, and loss of their hopes for and future relationship with the dying person

 C. Mourning

  1. The outward, social, public expression of a loss[5,6]

  2. Are influenced greatly by religious and cultural practices[1, 5]

  3. Mourning practices in the United States include publishing an obituary notice in the newspaper, having visitation opportunities for friends and families, conducting a funeral or memorial service

  4. Such public expressions of feelings (mourning) helps the person move towards healing[5]

 D. Bereavement

  1. The state or situation of having experienced the death of a loved one[3]

  2. Includes both grief (the inward feelings caused by the loss) and mourning (the outward behaviors that are more obvious to others)

III. Normal Responses to Grief [2,3,5]

 A. Physical

  1. Lack of energy, feeling tired or weak

  2. Chest pain or tightness

  3. Shortness of breath

  4. Dryness or lump in throat

  5. Stomach aches

  6. Nausea

  7. Problems with sleep

  8. Headaches

  9. Lack of appetite, weight loss

  10. Dizziness

  11. Frequent colds or other illness

> *Normal responses to grief can be:*
>
> ❖ *Physical*
> ❖ *Emotional*
> ❖ *Spiritual*

12. Feeling of hollowness in the stomach

13. Sensitivity to noise

14. Irritability, extreme tension

15. Muscle weakness, shaking, trembling

B. Cognitive (having to do with thoughts or thinking ability)

1. Confusion

2. Inability to concentrate

3. Disbelief or denial that loss has occurred

4. Constant thinking about the deceased

5. Feeling that the deceased is present

6. Hearing or seeing the deceased

7. Memory loss

8. Slow responses to questions

9. Dreaming about the deceased

C. Emotional (having to do with feelings)

1. Sadness

2. Anxiety

3. Feelings of guilt or shame

4. Anger

5. Relief or sense of peace

6. Loss of interest in usual activities

7. Numbness, lack of feeling

8. Sense of hopelessness

9. Mood swings

10. Apathy (lack of feeling or concern about anything)

11. Fearfulness, worrying

D. Behaviors

1. Crying

2. Withdrawing, wanting to be alone

3. Over-reacting to things or events

4. Unable to work, not productive at work

5. Changes in sleep patterns

6. Acting like the deceased

7. Visiting places or carrying things that belonged to the deceased

8. Drinking too much alcohol

9. Abusing medications; e.g., taking tranquilizers or sleeping pills to escape the pain of grief

E. Spiritual responses: may be similar to the emotional response, and include

1. Doubting that God exists or anger with God

2. Loss of hope

3. Inability to find meaning in life

F. Experiencing any combination of the above feelings and behaviors is normal after a loss
   1. Most persons will gradually get back to more normal functioning
   2. It is only when these feelings, thoughts, and behaviors go on for long periods and continue to interfere with normal life that they are a serious problem

IV. Factors that affect how someone grieves[2]

A. How he or she was related to the person mourning, e.g., a person will likely react differently to the death of a child or spouse than to the death of an elderly parent
B. The type of relationship the person had with the deceased
   1. How close the person was to the deceased
   2. How strong or positive the feelings towards that person are
   3. Any conflicts between the bereaved person and the deceased
   4. How much the bereaved person depended on the person who died
C. How the person died
   1. Where the death occurred
   2. Whether the death was expected or sudden
   3. Whether the death was traumatic or violent
   4. Whether the death was preventable
   5. Whether there were multiple deaths affecting the bereaved person
D. What previous losses the bereaved person experienced and how they coped with those losses
   1. A person will grieve differently if it is the first significant loss they have experienced
   2. A person who has experienced many losses may be overcome by their feelings or they may have learned to cope well
E. The type of person the bereaved is
   1. Age
      a) Children grieve differently depending on their age
      b) Young people have different feelings and needs than older people when grieving
   2. Gender
      a) Men often feel they must be strong and not show emotion
      b) Women are more likely to express their emotions openly and talk to others about how they feel
   3. People tend to handle their grief as they do other life problem, e.g., if a person is usually positive and hopeful, they will often have an easier recovery from the grief but a person who tends to be negative may have a more difficult time with the grieving process
   4. Beliefs, culture, and values: spiritual beliefs and religious and cultural practices may help the person during the grieving period
F. Social support
   1. People with good support from family and friends usually have an easier time getting over a loss
   2. People who belong to organizations, clubs or to a church tend to have more support available

G. Other stressors or problems: if a person is having other problems such as losing a job or financial difficulties, it affects how he or she grieves

V. Stages or Tasks of Grief

A. Many of those who have studied grieving people believe that the grieving person passes through a number of stages or tasks as they recover from a loss

1. Two well known theories are those of Elizabeth Kubler-Ross and William Worden

2. Persons may move back and forth through the stages or tasks of grief, and some never complete all

B. Kubler-Ross' five stages of death and dying[7,8] - these stages are often observed in persons who are dying as well as in their loved ones

1. Denial: the person does not believe the death will or has occurred

   a) The patient may deny that their illness is serious or will result in death

   b) The family may deny that the patient is seriously ill or a bereaved person may not accept that their loved one is actually dead

2. Anger: the grieving person becomes angry about what is happening or has happened

   a) This anger may be directed outward towards God for letting it happen, or towards the healthcare team or loved ones for their inability to make things better

   b) Anger also can be directed inward, with the dying person feeling anger at him or herself for previous actions, leading to self-blame and guilt

3. Bargaining: the grieving person may try to bargain with God or other people hoping it will change the situation e.g.,

   a) A smoker with lung cancer may promise to quit if their cancer will be cured

   b) A previously unkind husband may promise to be nice to his wife if she will only be allowed to live

4. Depression: as the reality of the situation sets in, the person feels the loss, and

   a) May be very sad and hopeless

   b) May cry or have trouble sleeping or eating

   c) May withdraw from other people

5. Acceptance: often, the patient, family and friends come to accept the illness and eventual death

   a) The patient may be at peace and able to talk with family and friends about dying

   b) The family may be able to make plans for the funeral and discuss how they will go on with life

   c) There may be times of sharing, laughter, and joyful memories

C. Worden's tasks of mourning[2] - these are the usual tasks a grieving person most complete to return to better functioning

1. Accept the reality of the loss: the person must first overcome denial and realize that the one they loved is dying or has died

2. Experience the pain of the loss: to overcome grief, the person needs to express the feelings and hurt that goes with it

   a) It takes time to deal with all the sadness and changes that a death causes

b) Grief is difficult work and the bereaved will need help and support from those around them

3. Adjust to life without the loved one: eventually the grieving person learns to accept that their loved one is gone and makes changes such as taking on new roles, learning new routines, or making new friends

4. Find a way to remember the one who died: although the grieving person gets better and returns to their activities and life, they never totally "get over" their loss
   a) It is normal and healthy for a person to find ways to remember the one that died
   b) The bereaved person may make visits to the cemetery, display photos of the deceased, or remember the deceased on holidays or special occasions
   c) Telling stories about the deceased loved one may be helpful

5. Life is forever changed when a loved one dies

6. Although these theories about how people grieve help us to understand their experience, it is important to remember that each person's grief is unique

VI. Children and Grief[1,4,9]

A. Children respond to loss according to age and maturity level

1. Infants
   a) Feel the grief of those around them
   b) Will notice changes in their schedules and the feelings of those who care for them

2. Babies from 10 months to 2 years
   a) Sense the moods of others
   b) Sense the loss of anyone who provides their care

3. Children between age ages of 2 and 5 years
   a) See death as temporary
   b) May think that the dead person is sleeping
   c) Will believe what is told them about the death as being the actual truth

4. Children between the ages of 6 and 9 years
   a) See death as final and real
   b) Do not have the coping abilities needed to deal with their loss
   c) May experience sadness, anger, guilt, fear, confusion and may be overwhelmed by their feelings
   d) May feel responsible for the death; e.g., "If I had only been more helpful, Mommy would not have died"

5. Preadolescents between the ages of 10 to 12 years
   a) Know death is permanent
   b) Are able to understand the rituals related to death (funeral, viewing, etc.)
   c) Know that the death has a serious impact on their family and themselves
   d) Realize that they will someday die

6. Adolescents between the ages of 13 and 19 years
   a) Understand death as an adult

  b) Are going through an emotional time in their lives and can react with intense feelings of fear, anger, guilt, and denial

  c) May show childlike behaviors

  d) May become depressed and withdrawn

B. Grief behaviors

 1. In younger children

  a) Nervousness or hyperactivity

  b) Excessive anger or acting out

  c) Nightmares, dreams about the loved one

  d) Worrying about death or health issues

  e) Separation anxiety (become upset when left by adults) or fears of being alone

  f) Being clingy

  g) Sleeplessness

  h) Not wanting to eat

  i) Change in personality

  j) Acting more childish or baby-like; e.g., resuming behaviors such as thumb sucking or bedwetting, which they had outgrown

 2. In older children

  a) Trouble concentrating

  b) Withdrawing from others

  c) Frequent illnesses

  d) Depression

 3. Extreme responses of older children and teens that need professional attention

  a) Sexual acting out or risky sexual behaviors

  b) Anti-social or delinquent behaviors

  c) Running away from home

  d) Experimenting with alcohol or drugs

  e) Talking about or attempting suicide

C. Helping grieving children

 1. Respond to children according to their age and understanding of death

 2. For an infant, provide a nurturing, calm environment

 3. Babies (10 months to 2 years) need extra support and love and should be held and comforted.

 4. Use words such as "death" and "died," instead of "gone," "passed away" or "sleeping"

 5. Try to maintain the child's normal schedule as much as possible

 6. Never lie about death to a child

 7. Young children need to be told about the death in a way that is calm and sensitive but honest

 8. Children should be told what to expect, e.g., changes in routine

 9. Children should be re-assured that the death was not their fault

 10. Encourage children to talk about the death and express their feelings

 11. They need love, understanding and support from adults

12. They also to be with their peers and should be encouraged to continue activities with friends of their own age
13. Teenagers also need encouragement to express their feelings
    a) Encourage them to be involved in carrying out responsibilities related to the death and helping younger siblings
    b) Their peer group may offer support and help as they grieve

D. General guidelines for helping grieving children
    1. Make sure they have opportunities to ask questions, express their feelings and receive the attention of loving adults
    2. Allow them to grieve according to their feelings and let them express their anger, pain, guilt, and sorrow so that they can adjust to the loss
    3. Allow the child to be part of the grieving process and participate in rituals
    4. Encourage them to be physically active and involved with their friends (acceptable time-off from grieving)
    5. Help them find support groups or attend camps or other activities for children experiencing a loss
    6. Art and music therapy may be especially helpful to children
    7. If problems continue or seriously affect their daily functioning, seek professional help

VII. Helping the Grieving Adult

A. Offer verbal support
    1. Helpful things you might say
        a) "I am so sorry"
        b) "What is this like for you?"
        c) "Tell me about your loved one"
        d) "What I remember most about your loved one is……"
        e) "What can I do to help you?"
    2. Things not to say: things that are not helpful
        a) "I know how you feel"
        b) "God needed your loved one in heaven"
        c) "This was God's plan"
        d) "You should not feel that way"
        e) "You will get over this"
        f) Do not give advice
        g) Do not try to make it better by saying things like "cheer up"

B. Use helpful nonverbal communication
    1. Smile
    2. Nod
    3. Touch or hug
    4. Listen quietly
    5. Accept periods of silence

C. Helpful interventions
    1. Provide a quiet, calm space for the family to grieve
    2. If you are present when the patient dies, clean and prepare the body for family members to view; allow family members to take part if they desire
    3. Arrange for the family and friends to be with the body as they choose
    4. Encourage expression of feelings and sharing remembrances about the patient
    5. Make sure that spiritual and cultural practices are followed
    6. Notify spiritual care providers (chaplain or clergy) if family desires
    7. Give emotional support: let the bereaved family know that their feelings are normal and acceptable; emphasize that each person will have a unique response
    8. Allow the bereaved persons to talk about the death and their role in caring for and being with the dying patient
    9. Respond to family members' requests for help
    10. Inform the family and friends of available bereavement services
    11. Send a note or card to the family
    12. Attend the visitation or funeral and express your sympathy
    13. Give the family member or friend a phone call several weeks after the loss to see how they are doing

VIII. Taking Care of Yourself

> *Realize that you experience your own grief as you care for people who are dying and their families.*

    A. Know and understand your own feelings about death and grief
    B. Realize that you experience your own grief as you care for people who are dying and their families
    C. Talk with your co-workers about your feelings and grief
    D. Ask for help if you are having a difficult time dealing with a patient's death. Many organizations provide supportive services to help staff cope with job related losses
    E. Involve yourself in activities that allow staff to express their feelings and personal grief such as memorial services and support groups
    F. Involve yourself in activities outside of work such as hobbies, exercise, and family events
    G. Take your vacation time and use it to get away from work and relax
    H. Be aware of "yellow lights" - behaviors that may indicate stress or grief, e.g., high levels of fatigue, overuse of alcohol
    I. If you are feeling very stressed and anxious talk with your supervisor and consider professional help

IX. Summary

    A. Grief is a person's response to a loss
    B. Mourning is the outward, social, public expression of a loss
    C. Normal responses to grief can manifest physically, emotionally and spiritually
    D. Grieving persons pass through a number of stages as they recover from a loss
    E. Realize that you experience your own grief as you care for people who are dying and their families

CITED REFERENCES

1. Jeffreys JS. *Helping Grieving People: When Tears Are Not Enough*. New York, NY: Brunner-Routledge; 2005.
2. Bozeman M. Bereavement. In: Kinzbrunner BM, Weinreb NJ, Policzer JS, eds. *End-of-Life Care:Twenty Common Problems*. New York, NY: McGraw-Hill; 2002:275-293.
3. Corless IB. Bereavement. In: Ferrell BR, Coyle N, eds. *Textbook of Palliative Nursing*. 2nd ed. New York, NY: Oxford Univeristy Press; 2006:531-544.
4. American Association of Colleges of Nursing (AACN) and the City of Hope National Medical Center. Module *7:* Loss, grief, and bereavement. *End-of-Life Nursing Education Consortium (ELNEC) - Geriatric*; 2008.
5. Worden JW. *Grief Counseling and Grief Therapy*. 3rd ed. New York, NY: Springer; 2002.
6. Burke BK. Loss and Bereavement. In: Ersek M, ed. *Core Curriculum for the Hospice and Palliative Nursing Assistant*. Dubuque, Iowa: Kendall-Hunt; 2003: 85-92.
7. Kubler-Ross. *On Death and Dying*. New York, NY: MacMillan;1969.
8. Head B. Grief and Bereavement. In: Ersek M, ed. *Nursing Assistant End-of-Life Care Education Program (NA-CEP)*. Pittsburgh, PA: Hospice and Palliative Nurses Association; 2006.
9. Kroen WC. *Helping Children Cope with the Loss of a Loved One: A Guide for Grownups*. Minneapolis, MN: Free Spirit Publishing; 1996.

Resources available at www.hpna.org

HPNA Patient/Family Teaching Sheet

❖ *Grief and Mourning*

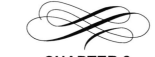

CHAPTER 8
SPIRITUAL CARE AT THE END OF LIFE

Barbara Head, PhD, RN, CHPN®, ACSW

Original Author
Barbara Head, PhD, RN, CHPN®, ACSW

I. Definitions

  A. Spirituality

    1. That part of the person, often known as the soul, which connects to a superior being, "higher power," or force, such as God

    2. Awareness of a divine presence

    3. Harmonious relationships or connections with self, neighbor, nature, God, or a higher being that draws a person beyond himself[1]

    4. May include religious beliefs and practices, but does not require that a person takes part in organized religion

    5. Beliefs and practices that give purpose, meaning and hope to a person's life

  B. Spiritual well being

    1. A sense of inner peace, compassion for others, reverence for life, gratitude, and appreciation of both unity and diversity[2]

    2. A sense that life has meaning

    3. Contentment that comes from feeling connected with something greater than oneself

> *Spiritual well being is a sense that life has meaning.*

  C. Religion

    1. An organized effort to express spirituality through rituals and specific practices, e.g., prayer, communion, baptism, fasting, and meditation

    2. These rituals and practices are connected with a set of common beliefs

  D. Spiritual care

    1. Team members' responses to a patient's/family's spiritual needs through various interventions, such as listening, accepting, and talking about life and its meaning, and coordinating care with the patient's religious community

    2. Efforts to help a patient have a feeling of spiritual well-being

    3. Providing opportunities for reconciliation or relationship with a higher power, such as God and self[3]

    4. Helping a person connect or reconnect to things, practices, ideas, and principles that give life meaning

II. Importance of Spiritual Care

  A. Spiritual beliefs affect how a person lives and dies

  B. Spiritual beliefs affect the patient and family's acceptance of hospice/palliative care

C. Hospice/palliative care is holistic; it deals with the physical, social, emotional, and spiritual parts of the patient and family

D. Spirituality contributes to quality of life for the dying patient

E. Spiritual beliefs and practices help the patient and family cope with terminal illness

F. Spiritual well-being has been found to contribute to a peaceful, good death[4]

III. Spiritual Needs of the Dying Patient

A. Give and receive love

B. Give and receive forgiveness

C. Find meaning and purpose in life

D. Life review, or telling the story of one's life

E. Develop hope that life can be lived fully and deeply

F. Develop hope for a life after death

G. Complete unfinished tasks

H. Mend broken relationships

I. Maintain positive relationships with God and others

J. Develop understanding of death

K. Take part in religious practices (prayer, Bible reading, meditation)

L. Accept oneself and be at peace

M. Die with dignity

IV. Signs of Spiritual Distress

A. Suffering or pain related to feelings of brokenness in one's relationship with God or others, loss of meaning and purpose, questioning of one's religious beliefs or values, or loss of inner strength and/or sense of well-being[5]

B. Person in spiritual distress may make comments such as[6]

1. "I thought I understood God; now I do not know anymore…"

2. "I feel so alone"

3. "How could this happen to me?"

4. "It is my fault I got the cancer. God is punishing me for being bad to my family"

C. When a person feels spiritual distress he or she may also feel

1. Hopeless

2. Depressed

3. Anxious

4. A desire for suicide or a hastened death

5. That she/he is a burden to others

6. A loss of the will to live

7. A loss of dignity or control

8. Anger towards God, clergy, loved ones

9. Confused or conflicted about beliefs

10. Uncertain about the meaning of life

11. Worthless

12. Extreme sadness

V. Spiritual Signs that Death is Coming Soon[7]
   A. Lack of interest in material things
   B. Less interest in talking about things that are not really important
   C. More silence
   D. Lack of concern for appearance (how one looks)

VI. Common Religious/Spiritual Views on Death and Death Rituals[6,8]
   A. The following information is general; not every member of each religion follows all practices and beliefs of a particular religion; always check with the patient and family to find out their particular beliefs
   B. Buddhist beliefs and practices
      1. Focus of most Buddhist practices is to attain a calm state of mind and to be compassionate
      2. Illness is a result of actions in this world or a previous life
      3. Healing results from knowing the wisdom of Buddha
      4. A temple or altar with a statue of Buddha may be in the house
      5. Frequent meditation or chanting
      6. Death is viewed as part of life and offers the chance to improve in the next life
      7. Some believe that the soul remains near the body for several days
      8. Family may ask that body be untouched for as long as possible so the spirit can make a peaceful transition to the next world
   C. Roman Catholic beliefs and practice
      1. Central focus is to obtain eternal life with God in heaven
      2. Illness may be viewed as punishment for sinful thinking or behavior
      3. Use of many signs or symbols such as the cross, the crucifix, holy water, statues of saints
      4. Going to confession and attending Mass are important rituals
      5. Praying is very important, may involve praying the rosary
      6. The ill may receive the Sacrament of the Sick
   D. Hindu beliefs and practices
      1. Death is natural and unavoidable, but is not actually real
      2. Do not eat beef, often practice fasting
      3. Physical modesty and cleanliness is very important
      4. Believe in many reincarnations before obtaining union with Brahman (God)
      5. Believe in four social classes (castes); person inherits his or her social class at birth
      6. Body is washed, anointed, and dressed in new clothes after death
      7. Body is cremated and water burial is preferred
      8. Only those of the same social class can touch the body
      9. Doing good deeds and giving to the needy are important
   E. Jewish beliefs and practices (content here refers to Orthodox beliefs. There are different levels of observance: Orthodox, Conservative, Reform, Reconstructionist, and Unaffiliated - each has different beliefs and practices)
      1. Focus on life and preserving it

2. Death is not to be feared as it is natural and comes from God

3. Soul exists before the body and continues to live after the body is dead

4. Kosher foods are eaten and should be made available

5. Sabbath is celebrated from sundown on Friday until sundown on Saturday; certain activities may not be allowed during this time

6. After death the body is not left alone until burial

7. Person's eyes should be closed immediately after death, preferably by the deceased person's children

8. Dead body receives a special washing by the Chevra Kadisha, specially trained members of the Jewish community

9. Burial occurs as soon as possible after the death

10. Death is followed by seven days of intensive family mourning; this period is called Shiva

F. Muslim or Islamic beliefs and practices

1. Patient may want to use remaining time for prayer and meditation

2. Members may follow strict dietary guidelines and period of fasting

3. Five periods of prayer are required daily

4. Believe that peace follows total submission to the will of God

5. Death is considered a natural process and a return to God

6. Cleanliness is important and may require bathing, cleaning at least five times per day before the required five periods of daily prayer; personal hygiene provided by persons of opposite gender may be very distressing

7. Body must be turned to face Mecca (the holy city) at the time of death

G. Protestant beliefs and practices

1. God is a holy being whom most Protestants believe exists within the Trinity of the Father, Son, and Holy Spirit

2. God is best understood through the Bible

3. God loves, protects, judges, and forgives those who ask

4. Believers have a direct and personal relationship with God through his son, Jesus

5. Focus on salvation through the gift of God's grace in Jesus' death

6. Belief in afterlife, heaven is promised based on personal salvation

7. Prayer, scripture, communion, and baptism are focal practices

VII. Providing Spiritual Care: Role of the Nursing Assistant

A. Be a good listener (also see Chapter 5)

1. Allow the patient and family to express their feelings, fears, and spiritual concerns

2. Do not rush the patient or family

3. Ask questions to encourage patient and family to talk about their beliefs, or lack of beliefs, but do not make judgments about what they say

4. Encourage the patient to review his or her life

5. Allow periods of silence and acceptance

6. Avoid imposing your own beliefs on the patient and/or family[9]

B. Develop a trusting relationship with the patient and family

1. Show an interest in patient's and family's feelings and beliefs

2. Show respect for the patient's and family's spiritual beliefs and practices

3. Validate the importance of the person's life

4. Let the patient and family know you care about them

5. Remain present with the patient through periods of fear and suffering

6. Know the patient's likes and dislikes and tailor your care to these likes and dislikes

C. Be aware of the patient's suffering and emotional pain

1. Such suffering may include regrets, guilt, failures, anger, feeling alone

2. Provide consistent, loving care

3. Recognize that physical symptoms often need to be relieved before spiritual needs can be addressed; for this reason, report any physical symptoms to the team and assist in treating them

D. Help the patient finish any unfinished tasks

1. Talk to your team about any such tasks you identify

2. If the team agrees, help with letter writing, making a phone call, or allowing the patient to talk through a relationship that needs mending

3. Encourage the presence of loved ones

4. Encourage the patient to discuss spiritual concerns with clergy or the chaplain

E. Know the patient's plan of care related to spiritual issues

1. If you have questions or concerns about the patient's spiritual needs or issues, talk to the team chaplain

2. Ask the chaplain how you can help with spiritual issues

3. Encourage and assist the patient with devotional activities (prayers, meditation, bible reading, etc.)

F. Be aware of your own spiritual beliefs and needs and become comfortable with your own spirituality so you can accept the beliefs of others

G. Provide a pleasant, homelike, peaceful environment including music, scenes of nature, flowers, etc.

H. Foster hope

1. Support the patient's and family's efforts to cope with the end of life

2. When appropriate, share feelings of delight, joy or humor

3. Help the patient set and obtain short-term goals

4. Reinforce the patient's accomplishments and successful coping

5. Allow the patient to make choices and maintain control

VIII. Summary

1. Spiritual care is the care provider's response to the patient's need to connect with a superior force or being and give meaning to life

2. Spiritual beliefs and practices are important to hospice and palliative patients and families

3. The patient's and family's spiritual needs include experiencing and communicating love, forgiveness, and acceptance; finding meaning and purpose in life, taking part in life review, maintaining hope, and peace

4. Various religions have different beliefs and practices about death and dying; one should always learn about the patient's beliefs and provide care according to those beliefs and related practices

5. Spiritual care includes being a good listener, encouraging religious practices and life review, respecting the patient's and family's beliefs and religious practices, developing a trusting relationship, encouraging hope, assisting with unfinished tasks, and working with the team to plan and carry out spiritual care

CITED REFERENCES

1. Taylor EJ. Spiritual assessment. In: Ferrell BR, Coyle N, eds. *Textbook of Palliative Nursing.* 2nd ed. New York, NY: Oxford University Press; 2006:581-594.

2. Vaughn F. *The Inward Arc: Healing and Wholeness in Psychotherapy and Spirituality.* Boston, MA: New Science Library; 1986.

3. Kemp C. Spiritual care interventions. In: Ferrell BR, Coyle N, eds. *Textbook of Palliative Nursing.* 2nd ed. New York, NY: Oxford University Press; 2006: 595-604.

4. Kruse BG, Ruder S. Spirituality and coping at the end of life. *Journal of Hospice and Palliative Nursing.* 2007;9: 296-304.

5. Villagomeza LR. Spiritual distress in adult cancer patients: Toward conceptual clarity. *Holistic Nursing Practice.* 2005;19: 285-294.

6. American Association of Colleges of Nursing (AACN) and the City of Hope. Module 5: Cultural and spiritual considerations in end-of-life care. *End-of-Life Nursing Education Consortium (ELNEC) – Geriatric;* 2008.

7. Kalina K. *Midwife for Souls: Spiritual Care for the Dying.* Boston, MA: St. Paul Books and Media; 1993.

8. American Association of Colleges of Nursing and the City of Hope. Module 4: Cultural considerations in end-of-life care. *End-of-Life Nursing Education Consortium (ELNEC) – Geriatric,* 2008.

9. McCurdy D. Ethical spiritual care at the end of life. *American Journal of Nursing.* 2008;108(5):11.

Resources available at www.hpna.org

HPNA Patient/Family Teaching Sheets

❖ *Managing Spiritual Distress*

HPNA Position Statements

❖ *Spiritual Care*

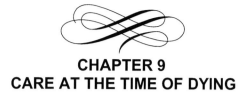

CHAPTER 9
CARE AT THE TIME OF DYING

Jeanne Martinez, RN, MPH, CHPN®

Original Authors
Jeanne Martinez, RN, MPH, CHPN®, Marianne LaPorte Matzo, PhD, APRN, GNP-BC, FAAN

I. **Introduction**

    A. Once it is determined that a patient is dying and treatment to cure the disease is no longer helpful, providing comfort care helps patient to have a peaceful death

    B. Nursing assistants can do much to make this time comfortable

    C. Care should be individualized to each patient's needs and goals

    D. Even very ill patients can be given control over their immediate surroundings

    E. Providing excellent care at the time of dying includes emotional support of family members and consists of listening and being present for people as they grieve the loss of their loved one

    F. The major ways to ensure good care to dying patients and to support their families is by

        1. Making the environment as comfortable as possible

        2. Giving care with an attitude of attentiveness, compassion, and concern to the individual patient and the family

        3. Working with the team to avoid any burdensome care, such as unnecessary weights, taking vital signs, or other care that may cause discomfort to the patient

        4. Respecting patient's and family's cultural, religious, and other values without judging them or imposing your personal beliefs

        5. Working as a team member by sharing observations, reporting problems and concerns, and supporting each other

II. **Patient and Family Needs and Goals Related to the Dying Process**

    A. Assist the patient to meet his or her end-of-life goals; ask patient the following questions

        1. Who does the patient want to be near him or her?

        2. What are the most important needs and goals for the patient before death?

            a) Prioritize care according to the patient's (then the family's) goals

            b) If there is conflict in what patients and family members want, patient desires come first

        3. Where does the patient want to die?

        4. Inform other team members about the patient and family's wishes and goals; it may take the entire team to work together to meet patient's goals, e.g., to arrange discharge and hospice services if the patient wants to die at home instead of in the hospital

B. Cultural influences (also ee Chapter 6)
   1. Determine important beliefs and values that affect patient's goals
   2. Respect the need for a patient to die on his or her own terms
   3. Avoid judging how family members cope with loss and death
C. Family needs
   1. Who is the patient's family or support system?
   2. Do patient and family goals conflict? Report conflicting goals and values to the team
   3. Assist patients and family members to "reframe hope;" e.g., help family and patients to meet short-term goals focused on hopes at end of life, such as hope to spend time with loved ones or hope to maintain dignity despite incontinence
D. Re-evaluation
   1. Continually reassess patient goals; help patients to decide what is most important to them
   2. Continually check patients for symptoms and whether medications and other interventions are helpful
   3. Always share patient's and family's wishes and concerns with the team

III. The Environment[3]

A. Physical environment
   1. Respect the environment as a sacred space, that is, as a place where a profound change is about to happen
   2. Individualize the environment; determine what is important and meaningful to the patient or family related to the following
      a) Objects and views
         i. What objects are meaningful to the patient or family, e.g., photos, rosary beads, books, pillows?
         ii. What should be in the patient's line of vision should he or she awaken?
         iii. What about window views?
         iv. Can the bed be repositioned to improve the patient's environment?
         v. If the patient is at home, is he or she isolated in a bedroom (and is that what they want) or is he or she in a central room of the home (and is that what they want)?
      b) Lighting
         i. Is natural light available?
         ii. Is room lighting harsh or gentle?
      c) Sound
         i. Is the room too noisy?
         ii. Does the patient respond differently to various noise levels?
         iii. Provide music, TV, other sounds that the patient likes, if that is what the patient wants
         iv. Vary the noise environment to enhance the patient's comfort, and sleep cycles
         v. Provide or increase calming sounds and decrease or stop sounds that disturb the patient

d) Family space in a facility
   i.   Can the environment be made less sterile or medical? Is it welcoming to families and visitors?
   ii. Are there comfortable chairs for family members and other visitors?
   iii. Is there a close common space for family members when they are not in the patient's room?
   iv. Are coffee, water, or other refreshments available nearby?
   v.   Is a phone available nearby, but outside of the patient's room, and a private place for cell phone use?
   vi. Does the environment promote privacy as much as possible?

B. Staff behaviors and attitudes
   1. Frequently visit the dying patient's room to check on patient status, comfort, and needs
   2. Maintain a balance between giving family members privacy and being there for support – ask what they need right now
   3. Sit down when talking with the patient or family members
   4. Listen carefully to the patient's and family members' issues; express your compassion and concern
   5. Stress may prevent family members from listening or remembering what you tell them; they may need the same questions answered more than once
   6. Recognize the importance of your presence, that is, being there rather than performing tasks; role-model this behavior for families and other staff

IV. Symptom Management Related to Decline in Status

A. Goals of care: watch for new or existing symptoms or problems; ask the patient which problems cause the most concern

B. Common symptoms in patients near the time of death (also see Chapters 2 and 3)
   1. Agitation/restlessness
      a) The person may make restless and repetitive motions, such as pulling at bed linen or clothing
      b) Observe for reversible physical causes, such as full bladder, constipation, fecal impaction, pain
      c) Moderate to severe restlessness could indicate terminal delirium, which may require medical management
      d) Consider that the cause of restlessness or distress may be emotional or spiritual in nature
      e) Nursing Assistant interventions
         i.   Speak in a quiet, natural way
         ii.   Lightly massage the patient's forehead, back, or arms, if acceptable to patient
         iii. Gently reposition for comfort
         iv.   Read to the person
         v.   Play some soothing music
         vi.   Try to decrease the number of people around the person
         vii. Avoid asking a lot of questions or talking a lot

viii. Do not interfere with or try to restrain restless motions, except to keep the patient safe

ix. Observe which actions or environment changes seem to increase or decrease agitation or restless

x. Report agitation and restlessness to the nurse and other team members

2. Pain

   a) Observe for moaning, restlessness, furrowing of the brow, and grimacing, which may indicate pain or discomfort

   b) Continue or begin non-drug pain therapies such as

      i. Gentle massage

      ii. Repositioning the patient

      iii. Pleasant diversions, such as music, being read to, etc.

      iv. For some patients, company and distraction can help pain, but for others a calm, quiet environment works better; ask or observe patients to determine what brings the most comfort

   c) Report patient report of pain or your observation of pain-related behaviors

3. Dyspnea

   a) Difficulty breathing, feeling short of breath

   b) Can be very distressing to patients and families

   c) Nursing Assistant interventions

      i. Positioning: put the head of the bed up; put pillows behind the patient's head; and if possible, sit the patient up in a reclining chair or position

      ii. Suggest that the patient move more slowly; keep still, lay quietly; and use pursed-lip or deep, slow breathing

      iii. Direct fan to the face or open a window (or both) to move air through the patient's room

      iv. Use relaxation or distraction techniques with the patient

      v. If the patient can communicate, ask which actions are most helpful

4. Noisy respirations or "death rattle"

   a) Caused by relaxation of throat muscles and pooling of secretions

   b) More disturbing to families than patient

   c) Nursing Assistant interventions

      i. Frequently change patient's position

      ii. Provide support to the families; assure them that noisy breathing does not mean the patient is in distress; avoid using term "death rattle" in front of patient and family

      iii. Deep suctioning is usually not helpful, and will cause more discomfort

5. Anorexia and dysphagia

   a) Anorexia: lack of appetite

   b) Dysphagia: difficulty swallowing

   c) Result of the process of the body "shutting down"

   d) Can cause the family distress; conflict can occur if the goals of therapy are not clear

e) Nursing Assistant interventions

    i. Offer conscious patients small frequent sips of fluids or bits of soft food, if the patient can sit up

    ii. Stop feeding if coughing or choking occurs, and report immediately

    iii. For unconscious patients, provide frequent, gentle mouth care

    iv. Help families to cope with the changes in patient status

C. General comfort care for patients nearing death

  1. Oral care

    a) Keep the patient's mouth moist

      i. Rinse the patient's mouth frequently with water or with swabs

      ii. Keep room humidified using spray bottle or humidifier

      iii. Apply lip lubricant generously to patient's lips

    b) Keep patient's mouth and teeth clean

      i. Use soft-bristled toothbrushes or sponge-covered oral swabs with non-abrasive toothpaste to brush teeth

      ii. Tongue blade wrapped in gauze and moistened may be used as an alternative to a toothbrush

      iii. Keep dentures and bridges clean; do not insert if patient has mouth sores

      iv. Avoid alcohol-based mouthwashes and lemon glycerin swabs because of drying and unpleasant taste

      v. Frequently rinse mouth; mouth rinses using, e.g., baking soda in water or saline rinses, chlorhexidine 0.2% (Peridex®)

      vi. Provide small chips of ice, frozen Gatorade™, or juice to refresh the patient

      vii. If the person is able to swallow, you can give him or her fluids in small amounts by syringe (ask a nurse for guidance)

    c) Use topical (applied to the skin and mucous membranes) anesthetics (medications that numb an area, e.g., Xylocaine®) for mouth sores

  2. Elimination management

    a) Use absorbent pads/adult diapers

    b) Apply moisture barrier to the skin

    c) Indwelling catheter for large amounts of urinary incontinence

    d) For fecal incontinence, assess for underlying causes, such as impaction, laxatives, and tube feedings

  3. Skin integrity

    a) Watch for skin breakdown, especially in bony areas, such as shoulder blades, elbows, heels, back of head, over the ears, and lower spine

    b) Prevent skin breakdown and discomfort through properly positioning the patient in bed and frequently turning the patient

    c) Be aware of the possible need to medicate the patient prior to turning her or him

    d) Anticipate the need for a special pressure mattress for comfort and skin breakdown prevention before patient declines; this action may reduce the need for turning the patient in the final days or hours of life

    e) Use a turning sheet for lifting and turning the patient

    f) If patient has skin breakdown

        i. Prevent further breakdown by carefully positioning the patient and frequently changing the patient's position

        ii. Observe the patient for pain or discomfort from the skin breakdown

        iii. Keep the area of the breakdown clean

        iv. Apply dressings as recommended by a nurse

        v. Control wound odors by gently cleansing the area, applying and changing dressings appropriately, keeping room well ventilated, and using room deodorizers if necessary

V. Psychosocial and Spiritual Issues

A. Psychosocial support for the patient

    1. Allow patients as much control over their environment and caregiving as possible

    2. Maintain patient dignity

> *Assume that the patient can hear all conversations; speak directly to the patient.*

        a) Assume that the patient can hear all conversations; speak directly to the patient, even if she or he does not respond

        b) Adjust language; e.g., do not use the word "diapers" rather use the term "briefs"

        c) Avoid speaking to others as if the patient were not present

    3. Be aware of possible fears commonly experienced at the end of life, e.g., fear of the unknown, of being abandoned, of being a burden to one's family or support system

    4. Communication/support

        a) Listen carefully and address the patient's concerns

        b) Orient the patient frequently, even if patient is non-communicative

        c) Periodically assess the non-verbal patient's ability to communicate by other means, such as squeezing hands or blinking

B. Psychosocial support for the family

    1. Listen carefully and address family concerns

    2. Allow the family as much control over the environment as possible

    3. When multiple family members are involved, be aware of who is the decision maker; consult with that person regarding changes and decisions about the patient

    4. Some families want to be present throughout the period when the patient is dying, whereas others are uncomfortable being near the person; respect individual preferences

    5. Common family fears at time of the death of a loved one[1]

        a) Being alone with the patient

        b) Patient will have a painful death; having to watch patient suffer

        c) Being alone with patient when patient dies and fear of their own responses

        d) Not knowing when the patient is dead

        e) Causing the patient's death by giving medications (in home care setting)

C. Grieving (also see Chapter 7)

    1. Grief is an individual, emotional response to a loss; is a process that is not orderly or predictable; begins before the death occurs and continues after the death of the patient

    2. The grieving person never "gets over" a loss, but can heal and learn to live with a loss and live without the deceased

    3. Nursing Assistant interventions

        a) Keep the family informed of the patient's status

        b) Prepare the family for what to expect as the patient becomes closer to death

        c) Provide information on grieving to help normalize the process

        d) If the family wants to, encourage them to participate in caregiving

        e) If family does not want to provide care or is emotionally or physically tired of care giving, give them permission to take a break and allow others to provide patient care

        f) Encourage families to talk with the patient before death

        g) Suggest that family members may wish to say good-bye when leaving the person, as death is unpredictable

        h) Provide resources for available bereavement support

        i) Provide spiritual support and referrals to clergy, as appropriate

        j) Respect the patient and family's spiritual beliefs. Never impose your own beliefs on others

D. Other Issues Around Dying[2,3]

    1. The "final rally"

        a) Days or hours before death, a non-verbal or comatose patient may suddenly awaken for a short time, be able to speak, or even eat a meal

        b) Behavior is temporary, but may confuse family members as to the patient's status

    2. Symbolic language

        a) Patient may talk about "preparing to go home," "going on a trip," "standing in line"

        b) Although the patient may seem confused, some healthcare workers see this as a normal process that they call "near-death awareness"

    3. Vision-like experiences

        a) Person may experience seeing or speaking to persons who have already died; he or she may also see places not presently visible to others

        b) This normal process may reflect that the person is detaching from this life and is preparing for death

        c) Do not contradict, explain, belittle, or argue about what the person claims to see or hear

    4. Inability of the patient to let go

        a) Patient may perform repetitive and restless tasks

        b) May indicate that something is still unresolved or unfinished and preventing the letting go

        c) May need to talk with the team who can assist you and the family in identifying what may be happening and help the person find release from tension or fear

        d) As hard as it might be, the family may need to give the person permission to let go

    5. Saying good-bye

        a) When the person is ready to die and the family is able to let go, saying good-bye is the final gift of love

        b) Saying good-bye achieves closure and makes the final release possible for the patient

        c) It may be helpful to encourage the family to hold or touch the patient and say the things that they want to say

            i. Message may be as simple (or as complicated) as saying, "I love you"

            ii. May include recounting favorite memories, places, and activities that were shared

            iii. May include saying, "I am sorry for whatever I have done to cause any distress or difficulty"

            iv. Family members may also want to say "Thank you" and "I will miss you"

            v. Tears and crying are normal and natural part of saying good-bye, express loss and sadness, and assure grieving people that there is no need to apologize or try to hide tears and sadness

    6. Dying alone

        a) Family members may have a goal of being at the patient's bedside at the time of death, and are upset it they are not present when the patient dies

        b) If this happens, gently explain this is not an uncommon occurrence – some people seem to die at the only time they are alone

VI. Death (see HPNA Patient/Family Teaching Sheet - FINAL DAYS)

    A. Signs that death is very near (hours or days) include

        1. Psychological and physical withdrawal

        2. Increased periods of sleeping

        3. Decreased consciousness

        4. Lack of eyelash reflex indicates deep coma

        5. Decreased and concentrated (dark) urinary output resulting from decreased blood circulation to the kidneys

        6. Skin coolness; hands, arms, feet and legs become increasingly cool

        7. Changes in skin color; paleness and sometimes presence of a bluish color resulting from decreased blood circulation

        8. Incontinence; control of urine or bowels (or both) may be lost as the muscles in those areas begin to relax

        9. Breathing pattern changes

            a) The person's regular breathing pattern may change and become irregular, e.g., shallow breaths with periods of no breathing for 5 to 30 seconds, up to a full minute, known as Cheyne-Stokes breathing

            b) Noisy respirations, death rattle

            c) Apnea, which is a period of no breathing

B. How will you know when death has occurred?
1. The signs of death include such things as
   a) No heartbeat or respiration
   b) Bowel and bladder incontinence
   c) No response
   d) Eyelids slightly open
   e) Pupils enlarged, do not respond to changes in light
   f) Eyes fixed on a certain spot
   g) No blinking
   h) Jaw relaxed and mouth slightly open
2. Ask the family "Do you know what to do at the time of death?" Talk with the family about what they should do if they are alone with the patient when the death occurs
   a) It is impossible to predict the exact time of dying
   b) Even though the death of a hospice patient is expected and is not an emergency, family and caregivers will still often feel "shocked" or "unprepared" when death does occur. This is a normal reaction to the loss
   c) Family (or you) should notify the team (hospice, on-call, or unit)
   d) In the home setting, the nurse will make the pronouncement and notify the physician and the funeral home
   e) In the home setting, the body does not have to be moved until the family is ready
3. Realize that even if the dying process is prolonged, you and the family may not be prepared for the actual moment
4. Aftercare rituals and family support
   a) Position the body (or assist nurse in positioning body) in an appropriate way for family viewing; if appropriate, remove oxygen tubing and other medical equipment
   b) Help, if appropriate, with any cultural or religious rituals that the family desires
   c) Encourage family to spend time with the body, saying good-byes
   d) Ask if other family, friends, or clergy needs to come to view the body before post-mortem care is performed
   e) Teach family what to expect
      i. Rigor mortis (stiffening of the body after death) occurs 2 to 4 hours after death
      ii. Air may escape lungs, especially when turning the body; assure family that this does not mean the patient is still alive
      iii. Bowel and bladder incontinence commonly occur following death
5. Post-mortem care: care of the body after death
   a) Handle the body with the same respect you would if the person were alive
   b) Clean body and groom as appropriate; in some settings, you might assist the nurse in doing post-mortem care, but in other settings, you will be expected to perform post-mortem care independently
   c) Ask if the family would like to participate in post-mortem care; some family members find it comforting to perform this last act of care for a loved one; in

some cultures and for some relationships (such as the death of a child), family participation in preparation of the body may be very important

    d)   Giving post-mortem care provides a good opportunity for you to say your own "good-byes" to the patient

    e)   Prepare family members for the removal of the body from the room or home; this is often a difficult process to observe and families may wish to say good-byes and leave the area prior to the body being removed

VII. Professional Coping with Care of the Dying

A.   Recognize the importance of professional coping and self-care

B.   Reframe your view of dying, so that death is an expected part of your practice

C.   Be aware of and explore your personal feelings about patients who die; find what works best for your coping

D.   Recognize your limits and ask for help when you need it

VIII. Summary

A.   Assist the patient to meet his or her own end-of-life goals (who, what, where)

B.   Enhance and individualize the environment

C.   Anticipate symptom management related to decline in status

D.   Anticipate psychosocial and spiritual care needs of patients and families

E.   Aid family grieving

F.   Recognize the importance of professional coping and self-care in working with the dying

CITED REFERENCES

1.   Martinez JM. Indicators of imminent dying. In: Berry P, ed. *Core Curriculum for the Generalist Hospice & Palliative Nurse.* 2nd ed. Dubuque, IA: Kendall/Hunt Publishing; 2005: 215-223.

2.   American Association of Colleges of Nursing (AACN) and the City of Hope National Medical Center. Module 9: Preparation for and care at the time of death. *End-of-Life Nursing Education Consortium (ELNEC) - Geriatric*, 2008.

3.   Callanan M, Kelley P. *Final gifts: Understanding the Special Awareness, Needs, & Communications of the Dying.* New York, NY: Bantam Books; 1992.

Resources available at www.hpna.org

HPNA Patient/Family Teaching Sheets

❖ *Final Days*
❖ *Self-care for the Caregiver*

HPNA TIPs Sheets

❖ *TIPs for Nearing Death Awareness*

CHAPTER 10
PERSONAL AND PROFESSIONAL DEVELOPMENT

Joanne E. Sheldon, MEd, MSN, RN, CHPN®

Original Author
Molly A. Poleto, RN BSN, CHPN®

I. Introduction

A. New and improved ways of caring for patients and families are constantly being developed

B. Nursing Assistants are required to meet the basic education and training requirements for their job and keep updated about new information and procedures

C. Professional responsibilities include such areas as

    1. Maintaining one's competencies (work skills) to a high standard of care

    2. Being an advocate for patients, families and nursing assistants

    3. Mentoring other nursing assistants

    4. Taking part in activities aimed at improving care for the dying patients and their families

    5. Modeling hospice's standard of care to all patients and families

II. Scope of Practice, Standards of Care, Competence

A. The Nursing Assistant *scope of practice*[1]

    1. Are the skills that nursing assistants are legally permitted to perform

    2. Is the distinct body of knowledge that directs the nursing assistant in providing hospice and palliative care

B. Hospice and palliative *standards of care*[1]

    1. Describe the basic skill level of care that should be provided to all hospice and palliative care patients and families

    2. Reflect the priorities and values of the employing agency

    3. Provide a framework for evaluating the nursing assistant's job performance

> *Nursing Assistant Resources*
>
> ❖ *Statement on the Scope and Standards of Hospice and Palliative Nursing Assistant Practice*
> ❖ *Hospice and Palliative Nursing Assistant Competencies*

C. The *competencies* for the hospice and palliative care nursing assistants [2]

    1. Include all the knowledge, attitudes, and skills the hospice and palliative nursing assistants need to provide quality care for seriously ill patients and their families

    2. Are measurable, meaning there is a standard way to evaluate a nursing assistant performance of a specific procedure, task, or behavior

    3. Include the following areas

<ol type="a" start="1">
<li>Clinical judgment in planning and providing care to patients and families to address their physical, psychosocial, and spiritual needs</li>
<li>Advocacy and ethics: nursing assistants uses ethical principles and hospice and palliative standards in providing care. Nursing assistants identify and advocate for patients' and families' choices and values (see Chapter 4)</li>
<li>Role performance: nursing assistants demonstrate knowledge, attitudes, behaviors, and skills consistent with the
<ol type="i">
<li>Performance standards, code of ethics and</li>
<li>Scope of practice of hospice/palliative nursing assistants</li>
</ol>
</li>
<li>Collaboration: nursing assistants encourage discussion with patients and families experiencing life-limiting progressive illness and bereavement to address their goals and work with the interdisciplinary team and community</li>
<li>Systems thinking: nursing assistants use agency and community resources to enhance quality of life for patients and families; systems thinking includes knowledge of and collaboration within the health and human service system</li>
<li>Cultural competence: nursing assistants demonstrate cultural competence by respecting and honoring unique values, diversity and characteristics of patients, families, and co-workers</li>
<li>Facilitator of learning: nursing assistants encourage learning for self, patient, family, other team members, and community through formal and informal education</li>
<li>Communication: nursing assistants demonstrate effective verbal, non-verbal, and written communication with patients, families, other team members, and community</li>
</ol>

<ol type="A" start="4">
<li>Other organizations that address general nursing assistants competencies
<ol>
<li>The Joint Commission</li>
<li>Community Health Accreditation Program (CHAP)</li>
<li>Accreditation Commission for Home Care (ACHC)</li>
<li>Agency/employer-required competencies</li>
<li>Center for Medicaid and Medicare Services (CMS)</li>
</ol>
</li>
<li>Competency evaluation
<ol>
<li>Definition: process where the nursing assistant is observed
<ol type="a">
<li>And/or tested on the performance of a procedure or on his/her knowledge about a certain aspect of care</li>
<li>Successful completion of this process is proof of the nursing assistant's competence in that procedure/area of knowledge</li>
<li>Example: hand washing. The nursing assistant washes his/her hands according to procedure while being observed by an evaluator. The evaluator documents the results</li>
</ol>
</li>
<li>Time frame: usually completed on a regular basis, such as annually and when new skills are required</li>
</ol>
</li>
</ol>

III. Professional Expectations and Development

<ol type="A">
<li>The nursing assistant *achieves and maintains competence* through
<ol>
<li>Education and training includes</li>
</ol>
</li>
</ol>

a) Initial nursing assistant training and nursing assistant certification as required by federal, state, and agency regulations

b) Continued education through in-service training for nursing assistants as required by federal, state, and agency regulations

c) Specific in-services and competency evaluation related to hospice and palliative care

d) Optional learning experiences to maintain expertise in hospice and palliative care

    i. Reading professional newsletters, websites

    ii. Viewing educational videotapes

    iii. Attending classes

B. The nursing assistant serves as a *mentor* for others

1. A mentor is an individual with advanced knowledge and experience who shares this knowledge with a newer team member; is available to listen, support, and guide the newer co-worker to become more familiar with their job duties

2. Experienced nursing assistants should mentor other nursing assistants in the work place and help plan and participate in in-services, orientation, and other educational programs

C. The nursing assistant takes part in *networking and fostering professional relationships*

1. Networking: making professional connections with other nursing assistants; provides opportunities to discuss similar problems and solutions; decreases feelings of isolation; occurs in many settings, e.g., at lunch, in the report room, at conferences

2. Nursing assistants should take part in organizations that promote quality nursing care such as Hospice and Palliative Nurses Association (HPNA) and volunteer for committees at work and for professional organizations

D. The Nursing assistant obtains *certification*[3]

1. Certification: the process through which a professional group validates a person's qualifications and knowledge in a specialized area of practice; involves meeting eligibility requirements and passing a standardized test that measures a national standard of knowledge needed to provide quality hospice and palliative nursing assistant care

2. Certification is voluntary, that is, it is not required by law for practice

a) Assists in meeting professional expectations by providing educational, networking, mentoring and advocacy opportunities

> *Certification is a process through which a professional group validates a person's qualifications and knowledge in a specific area of practice.*

3. Certification as a Hospice and Palliative Nursing Assistant (CHPNA™) is available through the National Board for Certification of Hospice and Palliative Nurses (NBCHPN®). For addition information about certification see the Candidate Handbook, available at www.NBCHPN.org

E. The Nursing Assistant is an *advocate* for patients, families, and team members

1. Advocacy is the process and act of representing the wishes, values, or concerns of another individual who may be less able to do so

2. Advocates must have knowledge of the person's wishes, etc., and be assertive in stating those wishes to others; they also must listen carefully to learn patients' and families' goals and values

3. The advocate always shows respect for patients and families even if there is conflict with them or the advocate does not agree with the patient's/family's values and goals

4. Nursing Assistants also must advocate for themselves and their fellow nursing assistants by reminding other team members and community about the important role of nursing assistants on the hospice and palliative care team; they also should support fellow nursing assistants when they have good ideas about improving care of the seriously ill and dying

5. Another way to advocate is to volunteer or join local or regional groups that focus on quality care of the seriously ill and dying

F. The nursing assistants *collaborates* with patients, families and other team members

1. Collaboration is working together with other people in a positive and effective manner where the combination of the knowledge and skills of each person in the group results in better outcomes for the patient and family

2. Requires open communication, mutual respect, and similar goals or mission

G. Each member of the interdisciplinary team contributes to the care of the patient and family by

1. Discussing what particular skills each team member possesses

2. Respecting each person's abilities

3. Respecting differences in skills and communication styles

4. Recognizing that the goal of the team is to help persons at the end of life

H. Ways to work together as a team

1. Share information and skills among all team members

2. Include patient and family as team members

3. Value each team member for his/her important role

4. Contribute to the care plan

5. Assist each team member in doing their job as necessary

> *Recognize that everyone on the team needs each other; no one is giving care alone.*

6. Identify team members with specific skills to work best with a particular patent and family

7. Help all members to be on "the same page" and identify goals of care

8. Actively take part in team meetings

I. Dealing with conflict among team members

1. Examples of things that cause conflict among team members

   a) Rivalry among team members

   b) Different communication styles

   c) Team members with differing goals and expectations

   d) Different personality styles

   e) Prior unsettled conflicts

   f) Job changes, job stress

   g) Lack of adequate staff or other resources

2. Techniques for resolving or reducing conflict

   a) Listen with understanding and without judgment

   b) Identify the issues

c) Seek help of supervisor when appropriate

d) Identify short- and long-term goals

e) Agree on one solution; record it as an agreement, if appropriate

f) Put solution into practice

g) Review how effective the solution was and readdress as necessary

J. The nursing assistant takes part in *quality improvement (QI)* and *research* activities

1. QI: a commitment and a systematic process to identify and solve problems with a goal to improve care and patient outcomes

> *Quality improvement is a commitment and a systematic process to identify and solve problems with a goal to improve care and patient outcomes.*

2. One model of QI is the Plan-Do-Check-Act (PDCA) Cycle

a) Plan: identify a problem, e.g., high rates of transfer to hospital shortly before death; design an approach to solve problem or improve outcomes, e.g., teach staff to talk with patients and families on admission about their wishes regarding hospitalization

b) Do: make the change and collect information about the effect of the changes, e.g., measure the percentage of patients who are transferred following the changes

c) Check: analyze the results; e.g., compare the percentage of transfers before and after the change - did they decrease, increase, or stay the same?

d) Act: if the changes resulted in better outcomes, then plan ways to keep the new practice going; if the outcomes did not change or got worse, develop different ways to approach the problem and test these approaches

i. Example, if staff education did not work, the agency could develop a formal procedure for discussing hospitalization with patients and families and charting their wishes

e) Research: a systematic study or examination of a problem or question; similar to QI, but usually more detailed

3. Nursing Assistants should participate in QI activities at work, e.g., by volunteering for the QI committee and offering ideas and feedback on agency processes and practices that could be improved; should also report problems that have (or could have) a negative or harmful impact on patient, families, and staff

4. Nursing Assistants could also volunteer to gather data and information as directed by the research team

IV. Addressing Professional Stresses Among Hospice and Palliative Team Members

A. Sources of stress

1. Your own grief

2. Feeling of helplessness

3. Sense that others do not care as much as you do

4. Lack of time to provide the care that patient needs

B. Manifestations of stress

1. Physical distress and fatigue

2. Feeling irritable a lot of the time

3. Emotional withdrawal from the persons you are caring for
4. Trouble with personal relationships
5. Starting to feel like you are the only one who can give good care
C. Interventions to prevent and decrease job-related stress
1. Recognize that everyone on the team needs each other; no one is giving care alone
2. Address your personal relations
3. Analyze your own emotional and spiritual needs
4. Find people whom you feel comfortable talking to and talk about your feelings and concerns
5. Practice healthy habits, e.g., eat a healthy diet, get 7-8 hours of sleep every night, exercise
6. Recognize that you cannot be or do everything for everyone: remember that even "Superman" is Clark Kent most of the time!

V. Recommendations for Professionalism
A. Accept responsibility for your actions
B. Complete tasks accurately and on time
C. Provide accurate information to patients, families, and team members
D. Accept criticism as a way to growth and self-improvement
E. Be flexible and open to learning new things
F. Be aware of your own limitations
G. Avoid being overly critical
H. Honor the wishes and values of patients and families even if you disagree with them
I. Work together with patients, families and other team members
J. Maintain an environment that is healing and supportive
K. Behave in a trustworthy manner; be dependable
L. Always dress and act professionally
M. Apologize to others, when necessary
N. Do not discuss personal problems at work or with patients
O. Provide care that is within your scope of practice; Follow the directions of the nurse to the best of your ability
P. Ask for directions and/or instruction if you do not know how to perform a task
Q. Maintain a sense of privacy for every patient when providing care

CITED REFERENCES

1. Hospice and Palliative Nurses Association. *Statement on the Scope and Standards of Hospice and Palliative Nursing Assistant Practice.* Dubuque, IA: Kendall/Hunt Publishing Company; 2002.
2. Hospice and Palliative Nurses Association. H*ospice and Palliative Nursing Assistant Competencies.* Pittsburgh, PA: Hospice and Palliative Nurses Association; 2009.

3. *Nursing assistant certification examination candidate handbook.* Pittsburgh, PA: National Board for Certification of Hospice and Palliative Nurses (NBCHPN®); 2008. Available at URL: www.nbchpn.org. Accessed January 11, 2009.

ADDITIONAL REFERENCES AND RESOURCES

American Association of Colleges of Nursing and the City of Hope National Medical Center. Module 6: Communication. *End-of-Life Nursing Education Consortium (ELNEC) - Geriatric Project*; 2008.

Center for Ethics & Human Rights. *Code of Ethics for Nurses.* American Nurses Association; 2001.

Fuzy J. *The nursing assistant's handbook.* 2nd ed. New Mexico:Hartman Publishing; 2007.

Stobo JD, Cohen JJ, Kimball HR, LaCombe MA, Shechter GP & Blank LL, et al. Project Professionalism, Philadelphia, Pennsylvania: American Board of Internal Medicine; 2001:6-29. Available at www.abim.org/pdf/publications/professionalism.pdf. Accessed January 11, 2009.

Schmidt TA, Adams JG. Professionalism and Ethics. Society for Academic Emergency Medicine: Michigan; 2002. Available at www.texaschildrens.org/Professionals/nursing/Toolkit/SAEM-%20Professionalism-Ethics.pdf. Accessed January 11, 2009.

Resources available at www.hpna.org

Position Statements

❖ *Value of Nursing Certification*
❖ *Value of the Nursing Assistant in End-of-Life Care*

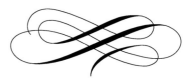

APPENDICES

APPENDIX A: CASE STUDIES AND QUESTIONS

CHAPTER 1
OVERVIEW OF HOSPICE AND PALLIATIVE NURSING ASSISTANT PRACTICE
Case Study and Questions

1. The focus of hospice and palliative care is
   a) Care for patients who are going to die within 4 weeks
   b) Providing therapies to cure a disease
   c) Patients with life-threatening illness and their families
   d) Helping people with advanced cancer cope with their illness

2. A "good death"
   a) Reflects the patient's and family's goals and values
   b) Occurs only in homes and hospitals
   c) Is not possible without hospice care
   d) Occurs when the patient is not given life-saving treatments

3. Nursing Assistants who provide hospice and palliative care
   a) Follow doctors' orders
   b) Must be certified by the NBCHPN
   c) Should not deal with the patient's spiritual needs
   d) Include certified nursing assistants working in nursing homes

4. Palliative care
   a) Involves a team that is always led by the physician
   b) Is the same as hospice
   c) Is focused on the relief of suffering
   d) Is not available if the patient is receiving hospice

CHAPTER 2
PAIN MANAGEMENT AT THE END OF LIFE
Case Study and Questions

Ms. Jackson is a 72-year-old patient with lung cancer that has spread to her liver. She lives in a nursing home and has two children who visit regularly. Ms. Jackson reports having pain in her abdomen that never goes away, like a toothache. An acceptable pain rating for her is 3 out of 10 and her current pain rating is 8 out of 10. When she gets out of bed, Ms. Jackson states the pain is "much worse" and "takes her breath away". She also reports that she aches all over at night and has burning pain that shoots down both legs, keeping her awake. Ms. Jackson's children report that she is more irritable when they visit. While you are talking to Ms. Jackson, you notice that she is frowning with every movement and clenches her fists every so often. However, she is pleasant and smiles often during your conversation.

1. Who is the best judge of Ms. Jackson's pain?
   a) The nursing assistant
   b) Ms. Jackson
   c) The doctor
   d) Ms. Jackson's family

2. It is important to tell the nurse that Ms. Jackson describes her pain as "burning" that "shoots" down her legs because
   a) These words suggest that Ms. Jackson has skin problems that need to be checked
   b) Ms. Jackson is having severe side effects of her acetaminophen (Tylenol®)
   c) Ms. Jackson is probably having nerve pain which should be evaluated
   d) Ms. Jackson's pain is exaggerating her pain to get attention

3. Ms. Jackson starts receiving oxycodone for her pain. Which of the following is **most** likely to happen now that she is taking an opioid?
   a) She becomes addicted
   b) She becomes constipated
   c) Her breathing becomes very slow
   d) She has trouble sleeping

4. What is the **most** accurate sign that the oxycodone is effective?
   a) Ms. Jackson reports that her pain is a 2 out of 10
   b) You do not see Ms. Jackson frowning at all during your shift
   c) Ms. Jackson's family visits more often
   d) At meals, Ms. Jackson is able to eat most of her food

CHAPTER 3
MANAGEMENT OF OTHER SYMPTOMS AT THE END OF LIFE
Case Study and Questions

Mr. Alfred Jerome is a 59-year-old patient with advanced lung cancer admitted to your hospice program several weeks ago. You are the certified nursing assistant from the hospice and have been visiting him three times a week to help with personal care. During your last visit, you note that Mr. Jerome is less responsive, and that his breathing sounds congested and noisy

1. What end-of-life symptom is Mr. Jerome having?
    a) Shortness of breath
    b) Fatigue
    c) Delirium
    d) Noisy breathing

2. What observation is the most important related to Mr. Jerome's symptom? If
    a) there is a suction machine available
    b) there are secretions in his mouth
    c) his oxygen is in place
    d) his urinal is within reach

3. After notifying the registered nurse of this change in Mr. Jerome's status, which of the following should you do next?
    a) Position Mr. Jerome on his left side with the head of the bed raised
    b) Be sure that Mr. Jerome has his urinal and call light within easy reach
    c) Provide Mr. Jerome with a hand and/or foot massage
    d) Reassure Mr. Jerome that this symptom will go away in a few days

CHAPTER 4
ETHICAL ISSUES AT THE END OF LIFE
Case Study and Questions

Mr. Day is a 58-year-old African American man with long standing diabetes and kidney problems. He is single and has one older brother, Henry, who visits him at least once a week. Henry's daughter, Louise, is Mr. Day's only other living relative. Louise is a nurse and has three young children, and visits her uncle whenever she has a chance. As a nursing assistant, you visit him twice a week to help him with his bath and personal care.

Two weeks ago, Mr. Day suffered a major stroke that left him unable to speak or swallow. He had never completed an advance directive, so there was no legally-named decision-maker. While hospitalized, Mr. Day's doctor urged Henry to agree to the insertion of a feeding tube to help Mr. Day maintain his weight. Henry wanted the feeding tube but Louise strongly disagreed. In the end, Henry went along with Louise's decision.

Today you arrive at Mr. Day's home and Henry is there. During your visit, Henry comments how bad he feels about the feeding tube. He states, "I cannot believe that I am going to let my brother starve to death!"

1. What is the <u>best</u> response you can make?
   a) "You were right to listen to Louise because she is a nurse and knows about these things."
   b) "Do not feel bad, this is what happens at the end of a person's life. They are not able to eat."
   c) "Would you like me to call the doctor and ask him to contact Louise again?"
   d) "What do you think your brother would want?"

2. During the team meeting, the social worker states that Louise based her decision on a comment that Mr. Day made to her: "I never want to be kept alive by any kind of machine. I am ready to have the Good Lord take me." In urging her uncle to refuse the feeding tube, what principle is Louise upholding?
   a) Nonmaleficence
   b) Autonomy
   c) Justice
   d) Beneficence

3. You find that it is hard to visit Mr. Day because you agree with Henry that Mr. Day is being starved to death. It is important to remember that
   a) these decisions must be honored even if you disagree with them
   b) you can urge Henry to contact a lawyer
   c) you can ask to be transferred from Mr. Day's care
   d) the healthcare team is letting this happen because they are racist

CHAPTER 5
COMMUNICATING AT THE END OF LIFE
Case Study and Questions

Mrs. Kerry is an 80-year-old Italian woman who is dying from pancreatic cancer. She lives with her husband and their oldest daughter, Anna. Mrs. Kerry is having difficulty eating and drinking. She also has pain in her abdomen when she tries to move or walk. In the past several weeks, she refuses to talk about psychosocial or spiritual issues to the nurse or spiritual counselor. Her family says that she has always been very quiet.

Jan, the nursing assistant, visits Mrs. Kerry three times a week to assist her with her personal needs. Today when Jan is helping her to bathe, Mrs. Kerry suddenly says, "I am going to hell when I die! I am afraid to die because I know that I am going to hell." Jan asks her why she believes that this is true. Mrs. Kerry responds, "Fifty-two years ago, I married my husband, but he was not Catholic. The church kicked me out because I did not marry a Catholic. I tried to live a good life, I am blessed with a great family and sweet husband, but I feel like I turned my back on God and He does not love me anymore. I chose my husband over God and He must be angry with me. I feel so guilty."

1. What is the <u>best</u> response Jan can make to Mrs. Kerry?
    a) "This sounds like it is a big burden to you. What can the hospice team do to help you?"
    b) Make no response because this is a personal issue for Mrs. Kerry
    c) Tell Mrs. Kerry's husband about the conversation and ask him if he ever considered becoming a Catholic
    d) "Mrs. Kerry, you need to talk to a priest about this. I am going to call Father Joe"

2. What nonverbal communication could Jan use during her conversation with Mrs. Kerry to show that she is listening carefully to what Mrs. Kerry is saying?
    a) Avoid eye contact with Mrs. Kerry because looking directly at her will embarrass her
    b) Lean away from Mrs. Kerry to give her space
    c) Cross her arms
    d) Nod her head while Mrs. Kerry is talking

3. Jan tells the team about her interaction with Mrs. Kerry. It was okay for Jan to share the story that Mrs. Kerry shared with her because:
    a) it made for a good story about someone dying
    b) it taught a very important lesson to anyone who listened to it
    c) the team needed to know what was going on with Mrs. Kerry to support her emotionally
    d) it proved that Jan was doing her job well

CHAPTER 6
CULTURAL CONSIDERATIONS AT THE END OF LIFE
Case Study and Questions

A nursing assistant is given the following report on a new patient he is to see: The patient is a 48-year-old male with end-stage lung cancer. He and his family moved to this country from Cambodia 8 years ago, and live in an Asian neighborhood that includes a large Cambodian community. The patient lives with his parent, wife and 12-year-old son. The adult family members wear loose cotton clothing while the son wears baggy jeans and a baseball cap worn backwards. The family is Buddhist.

When providing personal care on the first visit, the nursing assistant notes that the patient is barely responsive. He appears comfortable, but his breathing is shallow, and a little irregular. The nursing assistant is careful to be gentle and respectful when giving care, as he thinks the patient may be near death. He tells the patient he will pray for him, and makes the sign of the cross when leaving the room.

1. The son's clothing probably reflects that
   a) The family is poor
   b) He is acculturated to the United States
   c) He is a gang member
   d) He is disrespectful to his elders

2. The nursing assistant offering to pray for the patient and his making the sign of the cross
   a) Indicates the he is not being culturally sensitive
   b) Shows that he wants the patient to go to heaven when he dies
   c) Is appropriate because the patient is dying
   d) Is okay because the hospice is associated with a Catholic hospital

3. The best way for the nursing assistant to learn about the family's cultural practices is to
   a) ask the hospice social worker
   b) ask the patient and family
   c) read a book about Cambodian culture
   d) ask a friend he knows whose is Cambodian

CHAPTER 7
LOSS AND BEREAVEMENT
Case Study and Questions

You are the nursing assistant that has been providing personal care to Mr. Howard for about five months. You usually visit him twice weekly in his home. His daughter, Martha Jackson, has been very loyal and has taken a leave from her job to provide care for her dad at home. When you arrive at the home, it is obvious that Mr. Howard is very close to death. The hospice nurse visited yesterday and told Martha that her father would probably die soon. Martha leaves the room to take a much needed break from her caregiving while you are there.

1. While you are providing care, Mr. Howard stops breathing. The best **first** action for you to take is
   a) Call out to the daughter to come quickly
   b) Call the hospice nurse on your cell phone
   c) Finish providing care and then call the daughter
   d) Call him by name to see if he responds

2. When you inform the daughter that you are calling nurse because her father stopped breathing, she begins crying and yelling, "No, I am not ready to have him leave me." Your best response is
   a) "Just be glad he is no longer suffering"
   b) "Calm down. It will be okay"
   c) "It must be very hard to lose your father"
   d) "Everybody has to die sometime. It was his time to go"

3. When you go to the funeral home during the visitation, Mr. Howard's daughter tells you she has not been able to sleep and she keeps thinking that she hears her father calling out to her. You know that
   a) She is experiencing an abnormal grief reaction
   b) She needs professional help immediately
   c) These reactions are normal shortly after such a loss
   d) She is feeling guilty about her father's death

4. Martha also tells you that Amanda, her four year old granddaughter, keeps asking where great grandpa has gone. She asks you what she should tell Amanda. Your best response is
   a) "Wait until she is old enough to understand death better"
   b) "Tell her that her great grandfather has gone to sleep"
   c) "Do not allow her to come to the funeral home as it might give her nightmares"
   d) "Answer her questions honestly in age appropriate terms"

5. One month later, during an interdisciplinary team meeting, the nurse reports that Martha called and stated she is very angry with the doctor because he did not offer her father more chemotherapy. Which of the following statements helps you to best understand Martha's feelings?
   a) Many doctors give up on patients with advanced cancer
   b) A grieving person often feels anger as part of the grief response
   c) The daughter needs professional help
   d) It is not unusual for family members to sue their loved one's doctor

CHAPTER 8
SPIRITUAL CARE AT THE END OF LIFE
Case Study and Questions

Ms. Naomi Rosenblum is a 55-year-old orthodox Jewish divorcee with a diagnosis of breast cancer that has spread to her bones. Although she has moderate pain and limited mobility, she seldom complains and is usually talkative and pleasant. Today when Jason, the nursing assistant, visits, Ms. Rosenblum is sitting with her face towards the wall. This is unusual as she is usually watching the door waiting for his visit. He also notices that her breakfast appears to be untouched. Jason places his hand on her shoulder, and asks if she is ready for her bath. She responds, "I just want to be left alone. I am tired of being a burden to everyone." She denies any pain and states she is not hungry when Jason asks if she wants more of her breakfast.

1. Which of the following is the **best** response that you could make to Ms. Rosenblum?
    a) "Okay, I will see you next week"
    b) "I will call your rabbi and tell him that you need to talk with him"
    c) "Do you feel that God is punishing you?"
    d) "Why do you feel like a burden today?"

2. As death nears, what spiritual tasks might be important to Ms. Rosenblum?
    a) Identifying the positive impact she made during her life
    b) Completing a will
    c) Praying the rosary
    d) Giving away her belongings

3. Weeks pass and Ms. Rosenblum is entering the last days of life. Knowing that she is an orthodox Jew, what can you expect to happen at the time of death?
    a) The body should not be viewed by people who are not Jewish
    b) After her death, her body will not be left alone until burial
    c) She will need to be buried on a Saturday
    d) All mourning rituals will be completed within 5 days

CHAPTER 9
CARE AT THE TIME OF DYING
Case Study and Questions

The nursing assistant has been caring for Mrs. May, a 75-year-old woman with colon cancer, at the patient's home for several weeks. Mrs. May was alert and oriented when hospice care started, but over the past 2 week has become progressively weaker, and is sleeping more hours of the day. When Mrs. May was alert, the nursing assistant helped organize her room and bedside so things were in place the way Mrs. May liked them. The nursing assistant would often end her visit by reading the top news stories to Mrs. May when she was unable to read them herself, as she liked to discuss current events.

Mrs. May's sister has arrived from Missouri to help care for her. She has expressed concern to the patient's husband that her sister is "starving to death" as she is not able to eat enough since she is sleeping "too much". Mrs. May's sister discusses her distress over this in front of Mrs. May, although she never talks to her directly. Mrs. May's sister also says she is worried that Mrs. May did not attend church in her later adult life, which is important to the family's religious tradition. The patient's husband now seems concerned about what his sister-in-law is saying.

1. How should the nursing assistant respond to this sister's concerns about how much the patient is eating and sleeping?
   a) Tell the sister that she could call the doctor and ask for a feeding tube
   b) Explain that this pattern of decreased eating and increased sleeping is typical for patients at the end of life
   c) Ask the sister to identify Mrs. May's favorite foods so she can prepare them for her
   d) Suggest that the family try to feed the patient soft foods such as yogurt

2. What should the nursing assistant report to the RN or other interdisciplinary team members about the sister's concerns?
   a) The sister's specific concerns, and apparent stress over the patient's care
   b) Mrs. May's weight
   c) The name of the pastor at Mrs. May's church
   d) The amount of morphine that Mrs. May is taking every day

3. What should the nursing assistant do to help the family provide the best care for Mrs. May?
   a) Suggest to the family that they let the hospice provide all the physical care because it obviously upsets them
   b) Remind the family that they need to call the RN when Mrs. May dies
   c) Tell the family that they can stop providing oral hygiene because it is no longer necessary
   d) Encourage family members to talk to Mrs. May, as if she were still able to talk with them

CHAPTER 10
PERSONAL AND PROFESSIONAL DEVELOPMENT
Case Study and Questions

During a weekly hospice team meeting, a debate begins about a patient, Mr. Kern, a 61-year-old man with severe heart failure. Mr. Kern lives alone but has a few friends and family who visit occasionally. He is very demanding and frequently calls the hospice office with complaints. Amy is the nursing assistant caring for Mr. Kern. She has been with the hospice agency only for 3 months, since her graduation from a training program. Mr. Kern has been insisting on getting a tub bath. The staff feels that it would be dangerous to get him into the tub because he is unsteady on his feet and gets short of breath when he moves around. During the last visit, Mr. Kern asked Amy to give him a tub bath. When Amy responded that she did not feel safe putting him in the tub, he cursed and told her to leave. Amy comments during the meeting that Mr. K is concerned that a sponge bath does not get him clean enough. As a result, he says, "When I stink like this, nobody comes to visit me." The nurse who made one visit to Mr. Kern responds, "Nobody wants to visit this guy because he is a first class jerk! It has got nothing to do with his smell!"

1. Which of the following is the **best** way for Amy to respond to the nurse's comment?
   a) "Mr. Kern told me that he really does not like you and now I can see why"
   b) Amy should say nothing because she has not been with the agency long enough
   c) Amy should let the social worker or chaplain respond because they have more education than Amy
   d) "I realize that Mr. Kern can be difficult, but he deserves the same respect as other patients"

2. What professional responsibility is Amy demonstrating in her response to the nurse?
   a) Advocacy
   b) Knowledge
   c) Clinical competency
   d) Networking

3. Which of the following actions should Amy take to address Mr. Kern's needs?
   a) Call Mr. Kern's family and ask them to visit.
   b) Ask the nursing supervisor to call Mr. Kern and tell him that he is not allowed to take a tub bath
   c) Ask the nurse to overlap her visit with Amy's visit so they can both assist Mr. Kern into the bath tub
   d) Ask not to be assigned to Mr. Kern again

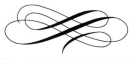

APPENDIX B: CASE STUDY ANSWERS

CHAPTER 1
OVERVIEW OF HOSPICE AND PALLIATIVE NURSING ASSISTANT PRACTICE
Answers

1. The focus of hospice and palliative care is

   a) Care for patients who are going to die within 4 weeks. **Incorrect** - Palliative care begins when a person receives the diagnoses with a life-limiting illness. Hospice care – because of the payment systems benefit – is generally provided to persons in the final 6 months of life.

   b) Providing therapies to cure a disease. **Incorrect** - Palliative care focuses not on cure, but instead the focus of care is on pain and symptom management and on psychological, social, and spiritual needs of patients and families.

   c) Patients with life-threatening illness and their families. **Correct**

   d) Helping people with advanced cancer cope with their illness. **Incorrect** - The focus of hospice and palliative care addresses the physical, psychological, social, and spiritual needs of the patients and their families who face *any* life-limiting illnesses.

2. A "good death"

   a) Reflects the patient's and family's goals and values. **Correct**

   b) Occurs only in homes and hospitals. **Incorrect** - A "good death" is possible in any setting, e.g., home, hospital, long-term care facility, prison

   c) Is not possible without hospice care. **Incorrect** - A "good death" is a death free from avoidable distress and suffering, reflects patients' and families' wishes and values. This can be accomplished by other care providers not necessarily "hospice care" though the hospice team has the specialty knowledge/experience.

   d) Occurs when the patient is not given life-saving treatments. **Incorrect** - A "good death" is a death free from avoidable distress and suffering, reflects patients' and families' wishes and values. Patients are taking a more active role in deciding what happens to them at the end of their lives; many people are choosing comfort care rather than high-tech intensive care when they have a disease than cannot be cured.

3. Nursing assistants who provide hospice and palliative care

   a) Follow doctors' orders. **Incorrect** - The nursing assistant is a valuable member of the interdisciplinary team and is supervised by the registered nurse

b) Must be certified by the NBCHPN®. **Incorrect** - The nursing assistant does not need to be certified. Though certification by the National Board of Certification of Hospice and Palliative Nurses (NBCHPN®) is highly valued and provides formal recognition of basic hospice and palliative nursing assistant knowledge. CNA (Certified Nursing Assistant), may be required in some states, facilities, or type of facility where nursing assistant work, e.g., long-term care.

c) Should not deal with the patient's spiritual needs. **Incorrect** - The nursing assistant is a valuable member of the interdisciplinary team that provides comprehensive caring for the whole person: physical, emotional, social, and spiritual needs.

d) Include certified nursing assistants working in nursing homes. **Correct**

4. Palliative care

a) Involves a team that is always led by the physician. **Incorrect** - Palliative care is achieved by using a team approach. The team come from many professional backgrounds or disciplines and together they make up the interdisciplinary (IDT team/multidisciplinary team).

b) Is the same as hospice. **Incorrect** - By definition, palliative care is the active total care of patients whose disease cannot be cured; instead the focus of care is on pain and symptom management and on the psychological, social, and spiritual needs of the patients and families. Hospice is part of palliative care. Palliative care starts when a patient is diagnosed with a life-limiting illness, whereas, hospice generally focuses on the patient with 6 month or less to life. The goal of hospice and palliative care is to achieve the best quality of life for the patient and their families when a cure is not possible.

c) Is focused on the relief of suffering. **Correct**

d) Is not available if the patient is receiving hospice. **Incorrect** - Hospice is part of palliative care. Palliative care starts when a patient is diagnosed with a life-limiting illness, whereas, hospice generally focuses on the patient with 6 month or less to life. The goal of hospice and palliative care is to achieve the best quality of life for the patient and their families when a cure is not possible.

CHAPTER 2
PAIN MANAGEMENT AT THE END OF LIFE
Answers

1. Who is the best judge of Ms. Jackson's pain?

    a) The nursing assistant. **Incorrect** - Pain is whatever the person experiencing it says it is, though people who spend a lot of time with the patient can provide valuable information to determine if the patient is in pain.

    b) Ms. Jackson. **Correct** - The person experiencing the pain is the best judge of pain. Pain is whatever the person experiencing it says it is.

    c) The doctor. **Incorrect** - Pain is whatever the person experiencing it says it is. The doctor may assess the patient and notice signs that may indicate pain such as changes in vital signs or non-verbal signs such as frowning or grimacing.

    d) Ms. Jackson's family. **Incorrect** - Pain is whatever the person experiencing it says it is. The family may report the patient is having pain because they do not want to see the patient suffer or they may not report the patient is having pain because they are fearful that it means the disease is progressing and the patient is getting worse.

2. It is important to tell the nurse that Ms. Jackson describes her pain as "burning" that "shoots" down her legs because

    a) These words suggest that Ms. Jackson has skin problems that need to be checked. **Incorrect** - This does not indicate specific skin problem, however it is a description of neuropathic pain.

    b) Ms. Jackson is having severe side effects of her acetaminophen (Tylenol®). **Incorrect** - This does not indicate a side effect of acetaminophen, however it is a description of neuropathic pain. Acetaminophen can be effective for mild pain.

    c) Ms. Jackson is probably having nerve pain which should be evaluated. **Correct** - This is a description of neuropathic pain and does need to be evaluated.

    d) Ms. Jackson's pain is exaggerating her pain to get attention. **Incorrect** - Generally patients at the end-of-life are exhibiting attention getting actions. They actually under report pain for fear the disease is progressing.

3. Ms. Jackson starts receiving oxycodone for her pain. Which of the following is <u>most likely</u> to happen now that she is taking an opioid?

    a) She becomes addicted. **Incorrect** - Addiction is a chronic disease when the person does not have control over their drug use. They use the drug compulsively, have drug cravings, and continue to use a drug despite physical and social harm. Addiction is uncommon in people with chronic pain at the end-of-life. Fear of addiction is not a good reason to discourage the use of opioids to manage pain.

b) She becomes constipated. **Correct** - Constipation occurs in most patients taking opioids and does not go away. To prevent constipation the doctor will order a laxative at the same time the opioid is prescribed. To further prevent constipation, encourage intake of fluids (water, fruit juices), fiber (fruit, vegetables), and encourage physical activity as the patient tolerates.

c) Her breathing becomes very slow. **Incorrect** - Clinically significant respiratory depression is extremely rare when patients in severe pain receive opioids and usually occurs at the start of treatment of with a major dose increase. Respiratory depression is defined as having a respiratory rate of less than 6-8 with decreased consciousness.

d) She has trouble sleeping. **Incorrect** - Troubling sleeping is not related to opioid treatment. Drowsiness may occur at the start of treatment or when the dose is increased and the patient should be monitored for falls.

4. What is the <u>most</u> accurate sign that the oxycodone is effective?

a) Ms. Jackson reports that her pain is 2 out of 10. **Correct** - Oxycodone (Percocet®, OxyContin®) is an opioid (pain medication) used to treat moderate to severe pain. The patients' report of pain is less using a pain assessment tool is an accurate measure of effective pain management.

b) You do not see Ms. Jackson frowning at all during your shift. **Incorrect** - Frowning may or may not indicate pain; therefore the lack of frowning does not indicate that pain medication was effective. Frowning can be a non-verbal sign of miscommunication, disagreement, or sadness; it is not a sign of effective pain management.

c) Ms. Jackson's family visits more often. **Incorrect** - Family visits are no indication that pain management is effective. The patient may enjoy family visits more when pain is relieved; however this is not the most accurate sign of effective pain management.

d) At meals, Ms. Jackson is able to eat most of her food. **Incorrect** - Appetite may or may not be affected by pain and pain relief. The patient may have a better appetit when pain is relieved; however this is not the most accurate sign of effective pain management.

CHAPTER 3
MANAGEMENT OF OTHER SYMPTOMS AT THE END OF LIFE
Answers

1. What end-of-life symptom is Mr. Jerome having?

   a) Shortness of breath. **Incorrect** - Shortness of breath (dyspnea) is difficult breathing or labored breathing.

   b) Fatigue. **Incorrect** - Fatigue is profound tiredness, which is unrelieved by rest, with a lack of physical and mental energy and weakness that interferes with ADL's.

   c) Delirium. **Incorrect** - Delirium is excessive restlessness with increased mental and physical activity most often caused by organ failure that cause chemical imbalances, but can also be caused or worsened by medication side effects, dehydration, infections, urinary retentions, stool impaction, lack of oxygen (hypoxia), tumors in the brain, or unresolved fears about dying.

   d) Noisy breathing. **Correct** - Noisy respirations are moist, noisy respirations caused by the pooling of oral and respiratory secretions at the back of the throat, with an inability to cough and clear the airway. This most commonly occurs in comatose patients. Though it is not uncomfortable for the patient, the families are often distressed hearing the "rattle" or the noisy respirations. Assure the families that the patient is not drowning or uncomfortable because of this. Repositioning the patient from side to side with the head of the bed elevated promotes drainage and can ease the noise. Reinforce that suctioning is not usually necessary and may even create more secretions. Avoid using the term "rattle"; use the words "congestion" or "noisy breathing."

2. What observation is the most important related to Mr. Jerome's symptom? If

   a) there is a suction machine available. **Incorrect** - Noisy respirations are moist, noisy respirations caused by the pooling of oral and respiratory secretions at the back of the throat, with an inability to cough and clear the airway. This most commonly occurs in comatose patients. Though it is not uncomfortable for the patient, the families are often distressed hearing the "rattle" or the noisy respirations. Assure the families that the patient is not drowning or uncomfortable because of this. Repositioning the patient from side to side with the head of the bed elevated promotes drainage and can ease the noise. Reinforce that suctioning is not usually necessary and may even create more secretions. Avoid using the term "rattle"; use the words "congestion" or "noisy breathing."

   b) there are secretions in his mouth. **Correct** - It is important to observe the secretion in the mouth and to report to the nurse in the event the secretions are excessive. Suctioning may be indicated if there is an excessive amount of secretions present which would be indicated by the patient drooling.

   c) his oxygen is in place. **Incorrect** - Oxygen is not indicated for noisy respirations. Oxygen may be helpful for difficulty breathing (dyspnea) or shortness of breath.

   d) his urinal is within reach. **Incorrect** - Having necessary items within the patients reach is always a practice however it is not related to this symptom.

3. After notifying the registered nurse of this change in Mr. Jerome's status, which of the following should you do next?

a) Position Mr. Jerome on his left side with the head of the bed raised. **Correct** - Repositioning the patient from side to side with the head of the bed elevated promotes drainage and can ease the noise that occurs with noisy respirations.

b) Be sure that Mr. Jerome has his urinal and call light within easy reach. **Incorrect** - Having necessary items within the patients reach is always a practice however it is not related to this symptom.

c) Provide Mr. Jerome with a hand and/or foot massage. **Incorrect** - Providing a hand or foot massage can be very calming and soothing for the patient however, it is not the next action.

d) Reassure Mr. Jerome that this symptom will go away in a few days. **Incorrect** - It is not correct therapeutic communication to provide false hope that distressing symptoms will go away. It is correct to providing support and reassurance to the patient and the family.

CHAPTER 4
ETHICAL ISSUES AT THE END OF LIFE
Answers

1. What is the <u>best</u> response you can make?

   a) "You were right to listen to Louise because she is a nurse and knows about these things." **Incorrect** - Louise, being a nurse, does not have anything to do with the decision. She is supporting her father's decision.

   b) "Do not feel bad, this is what happens at the end of a person's life. They are not able to eat." **Correct** - It may be reassuring to provide this information and reinforce that this does not cause the patient any discomfort. You can show Henry actions that he can do to provide his brother with comfort measures, such as providing mouth care, applying lip balm, sitting with and talking to him, etc.

   c) "Would you like me to call the doctor and ask him to contact Louise again?" **Incorrect** - This is not an appropriate action for you to take. Louise is supporting her father's decision. Ethical dilemmas can cause distress for healthcare workers and can be dealt by the entire team. If you feel distress over an ethical issue at work, talk with your supervisor.

   d) "What do you think your brother would want?" **Incorrect** - Louise is supporting her father's decision. Ethical dilemmas can cause distress for different members of the family. You are to report this to the team.

2. During the team meeting, the social worker states that Louise based her decision on a comment that Mr. Day made to her: "I never want to be kept alive by any kind of machine. I am ready to have the Good Lord take me." In urging her uncle to refuse the feeding tube, what principle is Louise upholding?

   a) Nonmaleficence. **Incorrect** - Nonmaleficence is not doing anything that is bad; do no harm; it is our obligation to protect our patients from harm. It is one of the main ethical principles (idea, concepts) used in healthcare to discuss and decide the "rightness" and "wrongness" of an action. This does not apply here.

   b) Autonomy. **Correct** - Autonomy is the supporting the right of the patient to make decisions and involves the patients right to choose. In healthcare this often means, that the patient may make a decision about treatment with which we disagree, but we accept and support the decision. Louise is supporting her uncles' decision. It is one of the main ethical principles (idea, concepts) used in healthcare to discuss and decide the "rightness" and "wrongness" of an action.

   c) Justice. **Incorrect** - Justice can mean respecting the moral and legal rights of a person. It is one of the mail principles (idea, concepts) used in healthcare to discuss and decide the "rightness" and "wrongness" of an action. This does not apply here.

   d) Beneficence. **Incorrect** - Benefiance is doing what helps the patient and prevents harm. It is one of the main ethical principles (idea, concepts) used in healthcare to discuss and decide the "rightness" and "wrongness" of an action. This does not apply here.

3. You find that it is hard to visit Mr. Day because you agree with Henry that Mr. Day is being starved to death. It is important to remember that

   a) these decisions must be honored even if you disagree with them. **Correct** - In healthcare the patient, and in many states the family, may make healthcare decisions on the patients' behalf about treatment with which we disagree, but we must accept and support the decision. Ethical dilemmas can cause distress for healthcare workers and can be dealt by the entire team. If you feel distress over an ethical issue at work, talk with your supervisor.

   b) you can urge Henry to contact a lawyer. **Incorrect** - This is not appropriate for you to do. Ethical dilemmas can cause distress for healthcare workers and can be dealt by the entire team. If you feel distress over an ethical issue at work, talk with your supervisor.

   c) you can ask to be transferred from Mr. Day's care. **Incorrect** - This is not appropriate for you to do. It may be difficult for you to understand and accept decisions that are made by the patient and/or family regarding treatments, however it is their decision and we are to support the decision and provide care to the patient. Ethical dilemmas can cause distress for healthcare workers and can be dealt by the entire team. If you feel distress over an ethical issue at work, talk with your supervisor.

   d) the healthcare team is letting this happen because they are racist. **Incorrect** - This is not an appropriate answer. It has nothing to do with ethnic issues rather the autonomy of the patients' decision.

CHAPTER 5
COMMUNICATING AT THE END OF LIFE
Answers

1. What is the <u>best</u> response Jan can make to Mrs. Kerry?

    a) This sounds like it is a big burden to you. What can the hospice team do to help you?" **Correct** - Many times the patient will tell you things they never told anyone before. They trust you. Communicating at the end of life is very important for the dying patient. It is important you listen to and assist the patient.

    b) Make no response because this is a personal issue for Mrs. Kerry. **Incorrect** - Dying patients often times have a need to talk or "clear the air" about something that happened in the past or that they need to say. You can provide non-verbal communication to Mrs. Kerry by nodding your head, sitting facing her and be attentive to what she is saying. Then you can ask her if she would like to talk with the chaplain. It is your responsibility to report this to the nurse.

    c) Tell Mrs. Kerry's husband about the conversation and ask him if he ever considered becoming a Catholic. **Incorrect** - This is not an appropriate action.

    d) Mrs. Kerry, you need to talk to a priest about this. I am going to call Father Joe." **Incorrect** - This is not an appropriate action. It is important to listen to Mrs. Kerry and report the information to the nurse.

2. What nonverbal communication could Jan use during her conversation with Mrs. Kerry to show that she is listening carefully to what Mrs. Kerry is saying?

    a) Avoid eye contact with Mrs. Kerry because looking directly at her will embarrass her. **Incorrect** - Non-verbal communication generally includes eye contact, however in certain cultures this may not be appropriate.

    b) Lean away from Mrs. Kerry to give her space. **Incorrect** - Non-verbal communication generally includes lean toward the person that is talking. Leaning away is a sigh of distance.

    c) Cross her arms. **Incorrect** - Crossing the arms generally indicate that the conversation is closed or the listening is bored. Is is not a sign of listening carefully.

    d) Nod her head while Mrs. Kerry is talking. **Correct** - Non-verbal communication skills for listening include; facing the person and maintain eye contact (except is certain cultures), nodding your head, murmuring "mmm", positioning yourself so you are "open" meaning arms are not crossed but folded on your lap or holding the persons hand if appropriate, and leaning in toward the person speaking.

3. Jan tells the team about her interaction with Mrs. Kerry. It was okay for Jan to share the story that Mrs. Kerry shared with her because

    a) it made for a good story about someone dying. **Incorrect** - This is not the appropriate rationale. It is important for all members of the interdisciplinary team to be knowledgeable of the patients' situation as the best end-of-life care can only be achieved using a team approach. Discussions about patients are to occur only with those involved in the care of the patient. It is a breach of confidentiality to discuss a patients' situation with others that are not involved in the care.

b) it taught a very important lesson to anyone who listened to it. **Incorrect** - This is not an appropriate rationale. It is important for all members of the interdisciplinary team to be knowledgeable of the patients' situation as the best end-of-life care can only be achieved using a team approach. Discussions about patients are to occur only with those involved in the care of the patient. It is a breach of confidentiality to discuss a patients situation with others that are not involved in the care.

c) the team needed to know what was going on with Mrs. Kerry to support her emotionally. **Correct** - It is important for all members of the interdisciplinary team to be knowledgeable of the patients' situation as the best end-of-life care can only be achieved using a team approach. Patient situations can cause stress for healthcare workers and can be dealt by the entire team. If you feel stressed over a patient situation, talk with your supervisor.

d) it proved that Jan was doing her job well. **Incorrect** - This does not prove the nursing assistant is doing her job well, however it is a responsibility of the nursing assistant and any member of the team to keep the other team members informed of the patients' situation. It is important for all members of the interdisciplinary team to be knowledgeable of the patients' situation as the best end-of-life care can only be achieved using a team approach. Discussions about patients are to occur only with those involved in the care of the patient. It is a breach of confidentiality to discuss a patients situation with others that are not involved in the care.

CHAPTER 6
CULTURAL CONSIDERATIONS AT THE END OF LIFE
Answers

1. The son's clothing probably reflects that

   a) The family is poor. **Incorrect** - There is no support that the family is poor. His dress indicates he is trying to adapt to the teen culture of the United States.

   b) He is acculturated to the United States. **Correct** - Acculturation is a process of adapting to another culture. People immigrating to the United States may give up a certain habits or practices that were common on their home culture and adopt habits that are common in the U.S. His dress indicates he is trying to adapt to the teen culture of the United States.

   c) He is a gang member. **Incorrect** - There is no support that this is gang related.

   d) He is disrespectful to his elders. **Incorrect** - This is not showing disrespect to the family. His dress indicates he is trying to adapt to the teen culture of the United States.

2. The nursing assistant offering to pray for the patient and his making the sign of the cross

   a) Indicates the he is not being culturally sensitive. **Correct** - Cultural sensitivity is an awareness of differences among cultural groups. It involves showing a respect for differences among cultures, based on knowledge and experiences with other cultures in order to respond to the unique needs of persons who are from different cultures. If the nursing assistant was cultural sensitive, the nursing assistant would know that offering prayers and making the sign of the cross is not appropriate when caring for a patient who is Buddhist. If the nursing assistant did not know what is appropriate asking the patient and or the family is an appropriate action.

   b) Shows that he wants the patient to go to heaven when he dies. **Incorrect** - This is not an appropriate rationale.

   c) Is appropriate because the patient is dying. **Incorrect** - This is not an action that shows the nursing assistant is cultural sensitivity to the differences of anothers' culture.

   d) Is okay because the hospice is associated with a Catholic hospital. **Incorrect** - This is not appropriate. Cultural sensitivity is an awareness of the differences of another's culture and being culturally competent is the ability to respond to the unique needs, beliefs, values of the person from a different culture not the type of facility where they are receiving the care.

3. The <u>best</u> way for the nursing assistant to learn about the family's cultural practices is to

   a) ask the hospice social worker. **Incorrect** - The best way to learn about the family's specific cultural practice is to ask them. It is important not to make assumptions about specific cultural groups. Team members may be able to provide you with information, however this is not the best answer.

b) ask the patient and family. **Correct** - The best way to learn about the family's specific cultural practice is to ask them. It is important not to make assumptions about specific cultural groups.

c) read a book about Cambodian culture. **Incorrect** - The best way to learn about the family's specific cultural practice is to ask them. There may be differences within a cultural group, therefore it is best to ask the patient and or family about their practices and beliefs.

d) ask a friend he knows whose is Cambodian. **Incorrect** - The best way to learn about the family's specific cultural practice is to ask them. It is important not to make assumptions about specific cultural groups. There may be differences within a cultural group, therefore it is best to ask the patient and or family about their practices and beliefs.

CHAPTER 7
LOSS AND BEREAVEMENT
Answers

1. While you are providing care, Mr. Howard stops breathing. The best <u>first</u> action for you to take is

   a) Call out to the daughter to come quickly. **Incorrect** - This would not be your first action.

   b) Call the hospice nurse on your cell phone. **Incorrect** - This would not be your first action.

   c) Finish providing care and then call the daughter. **Incorrect** - This would not be your first action.

   d) Call him by name to see if he responds. **Correct** - This would be your first action to determine if Mr. Howard is responsive. As with any changes in a patients condition you would contact the nurse.

2. When you inform the daughter that you are calling nurse because her father stopped breathing, she begins crying and yelling, "No, I am not ready to have him leave me." Your best response is

   a) "Just be glad he is no longer suffering." **Incorrect** - This is not an appropriate response. It is best to encourage the bereaved to talk.

   b) "Calm down. It will be okay. " **Incorrect** - This is not an appropriate response. This is not therapeutic communication. You cannot say that it will be OK. It is best to encourage the bereaved to talk.

   c) "It must be very hard to lose your father." **Correct** - This response is encouraging the thoughts and feelings of the daughter.

   d) "Everybody has to die sometime. It was his time to go." **Incorrect** - This is not an appropriate response. It is best to encourage the bereaved to talk.

3. When you go to the funeral home during the visitation, Mr. Howard's daughter tells you she has not been able to sleep and she keeps thinking that she hears her father calling out to her. You know that

   a) She is experiencing an abnormal grief reaction. **Incorrect** - This is not considered abnormal. These reactions are normal considering the recent loss. Intense grief reactions that last longer than a year are considered abnormal. They are more likely to follow death from trauma, suicide or murder; occur if the bereaved experience many losses in a short period of time; have unresolved issues with the deceased; lack the supportive network of friends, care providers, and family; may involve server reactions and self-destructive behavior.

   b) She needs professional help immediately. **Incorrect** - This is not considered an abnormal reaction based on the recent loss of her father.

c) These reactions are normal shortly after such a loss. **Correct** - Grief is a process that begins before the actual death and continues among the survivors following the death; it is a normal response to loss; differs greatly from person to person; is personal (no one knows how anyone else feels when that person has had a loss, not even when the losses seem identical); and allows people to heal from the loss. The bereaved person moves through stages of the grieving process; Shock (denial and numbness because the loss has occurred); Experience the loss (feelings of anger or guilt); Reintegration (begin to live successfully without the departed). Intense grief reactions that last longer than a year are considered abnormal.

d) She is feeling guilty about her father's death. **Incorrect** - This is not an indication that she is feeling guilty about her fathers death.

4. Martha also tells you that Amanda, her four year old granddaughter, keeps asking where great grandpa has gone. She asks you what she should tell Amanda. Your best response is

a) "Wait until she is old enough to understand death better." **Incorrect** - It is not necessary to wait until the child is older. Communication with the child needs to be honest, using age appropriate wording and answer the child's questions honestly.

b) "Tell her that her great grandfather has gone to sleep." **Incorrect** - Using words of death and died instead of "gone" or "passed away" or "sleeping" is the appropriate approach when working with grieving children.

c) "Do not allow her to come to the funeral home as it might give her nightmares." **Incorrect** - This is not an appropriate action to take. Approaches to take with children include; never to lie to the child about the death; use words of death and died instead of "gone" or "passed away" or "sleeping;" give the child a chance to talk about the loss; and answer questions from the child honestly.

d) "Answer her questions honestly in age appropriate terms." **Correct** - Children's expression of grief is determined by age and developmental level. Approaches to take with children include; never to lie to the child about the death; use words of death and died instead of "gone" or "passed away" or "sleeping;" give the child a chance to talk about the loss; and answer questions from the child honestly.

5. One month later, during an interdisciplinary team meeting, the nurse reports that Martha called and stated she is very angry with the doctor because he did not offer her father more chemotherapy. Which of the following statements helps you to best understand Martha's feelings?

a) Many doctors give up on patients with advanced cancer. **Incorrect** - This does not help you understand Martha's feeling.

b) A grieving person often feels anger as part of the grief response. **Correct** - This is a normal grief response. Grief is a process that begins before the actual death and continues among the survivors following the death; it is a normal response to loss; differs greatly from person to person; is personal (no one knows how anyone else feels when that person has had a loss, not even when the losses seem identical); and allows people to heal from the loss. The bereaved person moves through stages of the grieving process; Shock (denial and numbness because the loss has occurred); Experience the loss (feelings of anger or guilt); Reintegration (begin to live successfully without the departed). Intense grief reactions that last longer than a year are considered abnormal.

c) The daughter needs professional help. **Incorrect** - This does not help you understand Martha's feeling.

d) It is not unusual for family members to sue their loved one's doctor. **Incorrect** - This does not help you understand Martha's feeling

CHAPTER 8
SPIRITUAL CARE AT THE END OF LIFE
Answers

1. Which of the following is the <u>best</u> response that you could make to Ms. Rosenblum?

   a) "Okay, I will see you next week." **Incorrect** - This is not providing support to the patient. It is the responsibility of the each team member to response to the patient's spiritual needs. Appropriate nursing assistant interventions include, being a good listener, developing a trusting relationship with patient and family by showing interest, compassion and being present.

   b) "I will call your rabbi and tell him that you need to talk with him." **Incorrect** - This is not the best answer, though the rabbi can provide support to the patient as it is the responsibility of the each team member to response to the patent's spiritual needs.

   c) "Do you feel that God is punishing you?" **Incorrect** - This is not an appropriate response.

   d) "Why do you feel like a burden today?" **Correct** - This response does provide encouragement to the patient to further express how she is feeling. This is an appropriate nursing assistant intervention as well as being a good listener, developing a trusting relationship with patient and family by showing interest, compassion and being present. Since this is a change in the patient's condition it is important to report this to the nurse.

2. As death nears, what spiritual tasks might be important to Ms. Rosenblum?

   a) Identifying the positive impact she made during her life. **Correct** - Spiritual needs of the dying patient include love, finding meaning and purpose in life, life review, acceptance, and peace.

   b) Completing a will. **Incorrect** - Though it is important to help the patient finish any unfinished tasks, this is not the responsibility of the nursing assistant. Completing a will should be completed earlier in the disease process.

   c) Praying the rosary. **Incorrect** - Praying is very important, however praying the rosary is not a practice of the orthodox Jewish faith.

   d) Giving away her belongings. **Incorrect** - This is not appropriate.

3. Weeks pass and Ms. Rosenblum is entering the last days of life. Knowing that she is an orthodox Jew, what can you expect to happen at the time of death?

   a) The body should not be viewed by people who are not Jewish. **Incorrect.**

   b) After her death, her body will not be left alone until burial. **Correct** - Jewish beliefs and practices related to dearth include the body is not left alone after death, the person's eyes should be closed immediately after death, preferable by the deceased person's children, the dead body receives a special washing by special trained members of the

Jewish community, burial occurs within 24 hours of the death (except no burials on the Sabbath) death is followed by 7 days of intensive family mourning (Shiva)

c) She will need to be buried on a Saturday. **Incorrect** - This is not correct. Burials do not occur on the Sabbath which starts Friday evening through Saturday evening.

d) All mourning rituals will be completed within 5 days. **Incorrect** - This is not correct. Intensive mourning for the immediately family occurs for a more extend period of time.

CHAPTER 9
CARE AT THE TIME OF DYING
Answers

1. How should the nursing assistant respond to this sister's concerns about how much the patient is eating and sleeping?

    a) Tell the sister that she could call the doctor and ask for a feeding tube. **Incorrect** - This is not a correct action for the nursing assistant.

    b) Explain that this pattern of decreased eating and increased sleeping is typical for patients at the end of life. **Correct** - The lack of appetite (anorexia) is a natural progression of the disease process and is a result of the body shutting down. It can cause the family distress, however it does not cause discomfort to the patient.

    c) Ask the sister to identify Mrs. May's favorite foods so she can prepare them for her. **Incorrect** - This is not a correct action. The nursing assistant can help the families care for the patient by providing gentle mouth care or small sips of fluids if the patient is able.

    d) Suggest that the family try to feed the patient soft foods such as yogurt. **Incorrect** - This is not a correct action.

2. What should the nursing assistant report to the RN or other interdisciplinary team members about the sister's concerns?

    a) The sister's specific concerns, and apparent stress over the patient's care. **Correct** - It is important to report any changes in the patients' condition as well as situations that may arise with the family or questions that the family may have regarding the care of the patient.

    b) Mrs. May's weight. **Incorrect** - This is not a concern considering the patient condition.

    c) The name of the pastor at Mrs. May's church. **Incorrect** - This is not the correct answer. This information should be in the patient files that are available to the interdisciplinary team.

    d) The amount of morphine that Mrs. May is taking every day. **Incorrect**

3. What should the nursing assistant do to help the family provide the best care for Mrs. May?

    a) Suggest to the family that they let the hospice provide all the physical care because it obviously upsets them. **Incorrect** - This is not an appropriate suggestion as it is important for family members to be able to care for their loved one if they wish, as well as it is important for the patient to have family members present.

    b) Remind the family that they need to call the RN when Mrs. May dies. **Incorrect** - This will not help the family provide the best care for the patient. If the family is alone with the patient at the time of death, they do need to notify the team (hospice, on-call, or unit).

    c) Tell the family that they can stop providing oral hygiene because it is no longer necessary. **Incorrect** - This is not appropriate. Mouth care is a general comfort measure. It should be provided for the patient. At the end-of-life the patient may be breathing through the mouth and the lips, tongue, and mouth can become dry. Gentle mouth care and applying lip balm is helpful.

d) Encourage family members to talk to Mrs. May, as if she were still able to talk with them. **Correct** - This is considered a psychosocial issue. Communication to the patient is important, even if the patient is non-communicative. Talking to the patient can comfort the patient as well as be comforting to the patient.

CHAPER 10
PERSONAL AND PROFESSIONAL DEVELOPMENT
Answers

1. Which of the following is the **best** way for Amy to respond to the nurse's comment?

   a) "Mr. Kern told me that he really does not like you and now I can see why." **Incorrect** - This is a non-professional and disrespectful comment.

   b) Amy should say nothing because she has not been with the agency long enough. **Incorrect** - It is the responsibility of each team member to be an advocate for the patient.

   c) Amy should let the social worker or chaplain respond because they have more education than Amy. **Incorrect** - It is the responsibility of each team member to be an advocate for the patient.

   d) "I realize that Mr. Kern can be difficult, but he deserves the same respect as other Patients." **Correct** - This is a responsible and profession response by the nursing assistant.

2. What professional responsibility is Amy demonstrating in her response to the nurse?

   a) Advocacy. **Correct** - Advocacy is the process and act of representing the wishes, values, or concerns of another individual who may be less able to do so.

   b) Knowledge. **Incorrect** - Knowledge is the familiarity or understanding gained through experience. It is the general awareness or possession of information, facts, ideas, truths, or principles.

   c) Clinical competency. **Incorrect** - Clinical competency is the process where the nursing assistant is observed or tested on the performance of a procedure about a certain aspect of care.

   d) Networking. **Incorrect** - Networking is the connections made between people of similar backgrounds that: provides opportunities to discuss similar problems and solutions, thus decreasing feelings of isolation.

3. Which of the following actions should Amy take to address Mr. Kern's needs?

   a) Call Mr. Kern's family and ask them to visit. **Incorrect** - This does not address the concerns of the nursing assistant.

   b) Ask the nursing supervisor to call Mr. Kern and tell him that he is not allowed to take a tub bath. **Incorrect** - This is not an appropriate comment.

   c) Ask the nurse to overlap her visit with Amy's visit so they can both assist Mr. Kern into the bath tub. **Correct** - This will provide the care that the patient needs and address the safety concerns.

   d) Ask not to be assigned to Mr. Kern again. **Incorrect** - This is not appropriate.